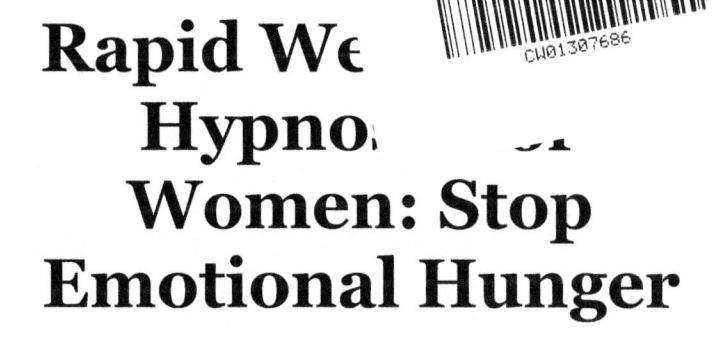

Rapid Weight Loss Hypnosis for Women: Stop Emotional Hunger

Guided Hypnosis for Women Over 40. Want to Burn Fat Fast? With Meditation, Psychology, and Affirmation, You Will Finally Be Motivated to Do It. Increase Self-Esteem and Stop Premenopausal Nervous Hunger.

Gerald Paul Clifford

© Copyright 2020 by Gerald Paul Clifford. All right reserved.

The work contained herein has been produced with the intent to provide relevant knowledge and information on the topic on the topic described in the title for entertainment purposes only. While the author has gone to every extent to furnish up to date and true information, no claims can be made as to its accuracy or validity as the author has made no claims to be an expert on this topic.
Notwithstanding, the reader is asked to do their own research and consult any subject matter experts they deem necessary to ensure the quality and accuracy of the material presented herein.

This statement is legally binding as deemed by the Committee of Publishers Association and the American Bar Association for the territory of the United States. Other jurisdictions may apply their own legal statutes. Any reproduction, transmission or copying of this material contained in this work without the express written consent of the copyright holder shall be deemed as a copyright violation as per the current legislation in force on the date of publishing and subsequent time thereafter. All additional works derived from this material may be claimed by the holder of this copyright.

The data, depictions, events, descriptions and all other information forthwith are considered to be true, fair and accurate unless the work is expressly described as a work of fiction. Regardless of the nature of this work, the Publisher is exempt from

Hypnosis For Easy Weight Loss: 2 Books in 1

Rapid Weight Loss Hypnosis for Women + Hypnotic Gastric Band: The Alternative to Surgery Is Your Mind

Gerald Paul Clifford

any responsibility of actions taken by the reader in conjunction with this work. The Publisher acknowledges that the reader acts of their own accord and releases the author and Publisher of any responsibility for the observance of tips, advice, counsel, strategies and techniques that may be offered in this volume.

Table of Contents

Introduction

Chapter 1: The Mind-Body Connection

What Is the Mind-Body Connection?

How Does the Mind-Body Connection Affect Your Life?

Common Mental Struggles That Manifest Themselves In The Body

   Childhood Trauma

   Covering Up Your Emotions

   Feeling Empty Or Feeling Bored

   Experiencing An Affection Deficiency

   Low Self-Esteem

   Low Mood

   Depression

   Anxiety

   Stress

   The Media

How These Struggles Can Lead People to Gain Weight

The Secret to Lasting Weight Loss

Chapter 2: Emotional Eating

What Is Emotional Eating?

What Is Binge Eating?

Why Does Emotional Eating Happen?

How to Tell if You Are Emotionally Eating

How to Read Your Hunger

The Science of Cravings and Food Addictions

Sugar Addictions: The Real Devil

How to Change Your Relationship With Food

Chapter 3: Addressing Your Current Mental State

What Are Core Wounds?

How to Address Your Core Wounds

- Journaling
- Self-Reflection
- Acknowledging Your Emotions
- Using Positive Self-Talk

What Is Positive Self-Talk?

How Can You Begin Using Positive Self-Talk?

Chapter 4: More Ways to Challenge Your Mind

How Self-Care Can Help

How to Practice Self-Care

Using Meditation

Meditation Techniques

What Is Mindful Eating?

The Benefits Of Mindful Eating

When and How to Use Mindful Eating

The Mindful Eating Technique

Chapter 5: Food-Related Changes to Begin Making

Making Good Food-Related Choices

How to Begin Making Good Choices Using Intuitive Eating

What Is Intuitive Eating?

The Benefits of Intuitive Eating

How to Make Intuitive Eating Part of Your Life

What Kind of Foods Should You Choose?

Electrolytes

Vitamin D

Chapter 6: Weight Loss

How to Achieve Weight Loss Without Using Diets

The Science of Weight Loss

How to Develop and Maintain a Healthy Diet Without Dieting

How to Shift Your Mind Toward Weight Loss

Chapter 7: Learning to Love Exercise

The Benefits of Exercise for Your Mental Health

How to Begin Using Exercise to Your Benefit

What Is Intuitive Movement?

Cardiovascular Exercise Versus Resistance Training

The Benefits of Other Kinds of Exercise

How Exercise Can Change Your Relationship With Your Body

The Importance of Sleep

Chapter 8: Using Affirmations

What Are Affirmations?

How Affirmations Will Benefit You

How to Use Affirmations

How to Come up With Affirmations of Your Own

Chapter 9: Hypnosis Techniques for Weight Loss

What Is Hypnosis?

The Benefits Of Hypnosis

The Different Levels Of Consciousness

The Conscious Mind

The Subconscious Mind

The 5 Levels Of Consciousness

How Can Hypnosis Help With Weight Loss?

Hypnosis For Cravings

Self-Hypnosis

Other Techniques

Visualization As A Form Of Self-Hypnosis

What Is Visualization?

The Benefits Of Visualization

How To Use Visualization

Visualization for Creating a Plan of Action

Visualization for Achieving Goals That You Have Set Out for Yourself

Chapter 10: Motivation

What Is Motivation?

How To Find Motivation

How To Maintain Motivation

Self-Judgement And How To Overcome It

How to Make Your New Lifestyle a Habit

Tips For Success

Conclusion

Introduction

Welcome to my book, and thank you for choosing it! There are many other books on the market, and I am glad that you saw something in this one that made you choose it.

This book is a comprehensive guide for people who identify as women or those looking to support a woman in her weight loss journey. This book is for people who are eager to learn all that they can about weight loss, hypnosis, and how these two important concepts come together to help people achieve their goals! This book is for anyone who has struggled with weight loss or doesn't know where to begin weight loss. It doesn't matter what experience you bring to this book. It only matters that you have taken the first step by reading the first page!

This book will delve deeply into various topics surrounding the psychology of body image, weight loss, and motivation. We will look at how you can control your internal self to accomplish anything and achieve your goals. This book aims to equip you with the tools to control your life and body and make changes for the better. Through reading this book, I hope that you find some peace and a sense of compassion for yourself, as bringing about change is not an easy task.

We will begin by learning about some of the situations and causes that lead people to become overweight by looking at the connection between your mind and your physical body. We will look at some strategies for getting in touch with your emotions and feelings to self-evaluate and determine what led you to where you are currently. This book's philosophy involves looking deep within to find the root causes and deal with the issues once and for all, instead of finding band-aid solutions like most books of this sort.

We will then look at hypnosis and how it can help you make changes in your life through various hypnosis practices. We will look at hypnosis and how it impacts the mind-body connection, and the science behind why it has been proven to work.

We will examine how hypnosis can be useful for weight loss and how you can set yourself up for success, especially if you have been attempting to lose weight unsuccessfully for some time. We will also look at visualization to increase the chances of success and help you with any goals you have set for yourself in your life.

Our next topic will be Emotional Eating, which is rarely discussed, but that cannot be left out of the narrative. By examining your eating patterns, you can determine whether you are an emotional eater, which will help you to better understand how to approach your weight loss plan.

After addressing the psychological side of weight loss and body image, we will delve more into the science of weight loss, weight loss techniques, diets, and exercise. We will look at how you can plan for yourself to work with your lifestyle to ensure success. Finally, we will look at how to put everything we have discussed together in the form of a plan and deal with setbacks or challenges that you will likely face along the way.

In the first chapter of this book, we will discuss the mind-body connection and how this may be presenting itself in your life. Be prepared for some self-reflection and realization, which is the first step in making any changes in one's life.

This book will delve into various topics surrounding weight loss and hypnosis, including but not limited to the following;

- The mind-body connection and how this plays a crucial role in your weight loss journey

- How to use affirmations and self-hypnosis to achieve your goals of lasting weight loss

- How to use meditation to combat food cravings and overcome food addictions (we all have them!)

- How to break free from the reigns of sugar cravings and sugar dependence

- How to lose weight FOR GOOD without the use of diets that make you feel defeated

- How to use the technique of mindful eating

- Essential techniques and strategies for using self-hypnosis

- Tips and tricks for finding and maintaining motivation to stick to your plan

- How to overcome binge eating and how to change your relationship with food

Without further ado, let's begin, but before moving onto the first chapter of this book, I want to give a brief disclaimer;

This book is not supposed to replace medical advice. It is not responsible for the actions or the results of the reader. Please seek out the advice of a doctor before starting any health program. The author is not a medical doctor, and the information in this book is meant only to supplement your health decisions and actions, not dictate them. Scientists are still researching the wonders of Autophagy at this very moment, even as I write this book. Please enjoy the information provided but also be wise in consuming it.

Now, let's get to the good stuff!

Chapter 1: The Mind-Body Connection

In this chapter, I will begin the book by talking about something called the *mind-body connection*. This idea may seem self-explanatory, but we will be delving into some pretty deep territory, so I will begin with the basics, and we will move on from there.

What Is the Mind-Body Connection?

This chapter talks about the *mind-body connection*, which is the term used to describe a concept that states that a person's internal or mental state (their thoughts, feelings, beliefs, etc.) can lead to physical, biological events, changes, or repercussions in the body.

How Does the Mind-Body Connection Affect Your Life?

You may be wondering how these two seemingly unrelated things (the inner world and the outer body) can be considered related. Over time, your body learns that eating certain foods (like those containing processed sugars or salts such as fast food and quick pastries) makes the body feel rewarded, positive and happy for some time after these foods are ingested.

When you feel sad or worried, your body feels this and looks for ways to remedy these negative feelings. Your brain then connects the mind's feelings with the reward that it knows that it can get from eating certain foods. As a result, eating these foods will turn its inner state from negative to positive and make it feel better.

As this process happens in your mind's background without you being aware of it, you then consciously feel a craving for those foods (like sugary snacks or salty fast-food meals) as a result. You may not even be aware of why you are craving them, as it all happens so fast in the subconscious mind. If you decide to give in to this craving and eat something like a microwave pizza snack, your body will feel rewarded and happy for a brief period. This process reinforces the concept believed by your brain that craving food to make itself feel better emotionally has worked.

If you feel down and guilty that you ate something unhealthy, your brain will again try and remedy these negative emotions by craving food. This process is how a cycle of emotional eating can then begin without you being any the wiser.

Because scientists and psychiatrists come to understand this process in the brain and the body, they know that the mind and the body are inextricably connected. Those food cravings or even being overweight can often indicate emotional deficiencies in emotional struggles.

For this reason, it is important to address the underlying issues when trying to lose weight or stop the cycle of emotional eating. By dealing with the root causes of the problem, you can stop it from reoccurring. If you simply try to follow a crash diet for some time without looking deep within to find the causes of the struggles you are having, the chances of falling back into emotional eating are very high. Therefore, it is necessary to address the root causes to end emotional eating once and for all.

Common Mental Struggles That Manifest Themselves In The Body

Now that you understand how a person's internal environment can lead them to fall into a cycle of emotional eating or seek food as comfort and eventually become overweight, we will look at some of the factors that lead people to develop a tumultuous internal environment.

Several types of emotional deficiencies or causes can lead a person to develop disordered eating, resulting in weight gain over time. We will explore some of these factors in detail in hopes that you will recognize some of the reasons why you may experience struggles with eating or with weight loss.

Childhood Trauma

The first example of an emotional deficiency that we will examine is more of an umbrella for various emotional deficiencies. This umbrella term is Childhood Causes. If you think back on your childhood, think about how your relationship with food was cultivated. Maybe you were taught that when you behaved, you received food as a reward. Maybe when you were feeling down, you were given food to cheer you up. Maybe you turned to food when you were experiencing negative events that happened during your childhood.

Another cause could be the relationship you had with your parents or the relationship to food modeled for you in your formative years. Maybe you grew up in an emotionally abusive home, and food was the only comfort you had. These reasons are completely valid, which was the only way you knew how to deal with problems when you were a child. The positive thing is that you can take control of your life and make lasting changes for the better now that you are an adult.

Any of these experiences could cause someone to suffer from emotional eating in their adulthood, as it had become something learned from an early age. This type of emotional deficiency is quite difficult to break as it has likely been a habit for many, many years, but it is possible.

When we are children, we learn habits and make associations without knowing it that we often carry into our later lives. While this is no fault of yours, recognizing it as a potential issue is important to make changes.

Covering Up Your Emotions

Another emotional deficiency that can manifest itself in emotional eating and food cravings is the effort to cover up our emotions. Sometimes we would rather distract ourselves and cover up our emotions than to feel them or to face them head-on. In this case, our brain may make us feel hungry to distract us with the act of eating food. When we have a quiet minute where these feelings or thoughts pop into our minds, we can cover them up by deciding to prepare food and eat and convince ourselves that we are "too busy" to acknowledge our feelings because we have to deal with our hunger. The fact that it is a hunger that arises in this scenario makes it very difficult to ignore and very easy to deem as a necessary distraction. After all, we do need to eat to survive. This necessity can be a problem, though, if we do not require nourishment and we are telling ourselves that this is why we cannot deal with our demons or our emotions. If there is something that you think you may be avoiding dealing with or thinking about, or if you tend to be very uncomfortable with feelings of unrest, you may be experiencing this type of emotional eating.

Feeling Empty Or Feeling Bored

When we feel bored, we often decide to eat or decide that we are hungry. This hunger occupies our mind and our time and makes us feel less bored and even feel positive and happy. We also may eat when we are feeling empty. When we feel empty, the food will quite literally be ingested to fill a void. Still, as we know, the food will not fill a void that is emotional in sort, and this will lead to an unhealthy cycle of trying to fill ourselves emotionally with something that will never actually work. This process will lead us to become disappointed every time and continue trying to fill this void with material things like food or purchases. This compulsion can also be caused because of a general feeling of dissatisfaction with life and lack of something in your life. Looking deeper into this the next time you feel those cravings will be difficult but will help you greatly in the long term as you will then be able to identify the source of your feelings of emptiness and begin to fill these voids in ways that will be much more effective.

Experiencing An Affection Deficiency

Another emotional deficiency that could manifest itself as food cravings is an affection deficiency. This type of deficiency can be feelings of loneliness, feelings of a lack of love, or feelings of being undesired. Suppose a person has been without an intimate relationship or has recently gone through a breakup, or has not experienced physical intimacy in quite some time. In that case, they may be experiencing an affection deficiency. This type of emotional deficiency will often manifest itself in food cravings. We will try to gain comfort and positivity from the good tasting, drug-like (as we talked about in chapter one) foods they crave.

Low Self-Esteem

Another emotional deficiency that may be indicated by food cravings is a low level of self-esteem. Low self-esteem can cause people to feel down, unlovable, inadequate, and overall negative and sad. This feeling can make a person feel like eating foods they enjoy will make them feel better, even for a mere few moments. Low self-esteem is an emotional deficiency that is difficult to deal with, as it affects every area of a person's life, such as their love life, social life, career life, etc. Sometimes, people have reported feeling like food was always there for them and never left them. While this is true, they will often be left feeling even emptier and lower about themselves after giving into cravings.

Low Mood

A general low mood can cause emotional eating. While the problem of emotional eating is something that is occurring multiple times per week, and we all have general low moods or bad days, if this makes you crave food and especially food of an unhealthy sort, this could become emotional eating. When we feel down or are having a bad day, we want to eat food to make ourselves feel better; this is emotional eating. Some people will want a drink at the end of a bad day. If this happens every once in a while, it is not necessarily a problem with emotional eating. The more often it happens, the more often it is emotional eating. Further, we do not have to give in to the cravings to be considered emotional eating. Experiencing the cravings often and in tandem with negative feelings in the first place is what constitutes emotional eating.

Depression

Suffering from depression also can lead to emotional eating. Depression is a constant low mood for months on end, and this low mood can cause a person to turn to food for comfort and a lift in spirit. This lifting feeling can then become emotional eating in addition to and because of depression.

Anxiety

Having anxiety can lead to emotional eating, as well. There are several types of anxiety, and whether it is general anxiety (constant levels of anxiety), situational anxiety (triggered by a situation or scenario) can lead to emotional eating. You have likely heard of the term *comfort food* to describe certain foods and dishes. The reason for this is because they are usually foods rich in carbohydrates, fats, and heavy. These foods bring people a sense of comfort. These foods are often turned to when people suffering from anxiety are emotionally eating because they temporarily ease their anxiety and make them feel calmer and more at ease. This calming effect only lasts for a short period; however, before their anxiety usually gears up again.

Stress

Stress eating is probably the most common form of emotional eating. While this does not become an issue for everyone experiencing stress, it is a problem for people who consistently turn to food to ease their stress. Some people are always under stress, and they will constantly be looking for ways to ease their stress. Food is one of these ways that people use to make themselves feel better and to take their minds off of their stress. As with all of the other examples we have seen above, this is not a lasting resolution, and it becomes a cycle. Similar to the cycle that I discussed above, the same can be used for stress. In the case of stress, instead of a negative emotion making you feel down, stress eating can make you feel more stressed, as you can begin to feel like you have done something you shouldn't have done, which causes you to stress, and the stress eating cycle ensues.

The Media

The constant exposure to media that we experience on a day to day basis can lead to a negative internal environment over time. If you are constantly seeing photos of people who make you feel inadequate, or people to whom you are comparing yourself, you can begin to believe that you are not good enough or that you will never measure up. These thoughts can be damaging and can lead a person to turn to food for comfort. This coping mechanism can lead them to feel worse about themselves afterward, leading to even more emotional eating.

How These Struggles Can Lead People to Gain Weight

As we have seen so far in this chapter, there are various reasons why people may develop a negative internal environment in terms of their thoughts, feelings, and attitudes. Over time, this can lead to changes in a person's physical body, such as weight gain. These changes are clear evidence of the mind-body connection at work. This emotional turmoil could be due to any of the reasons I previously mentioned, such as stress or childhood trauma, and it can begin to cause a person to seek food as a means of comfort. If this is done over a prolonged period, it can lead a person to gain weight steadily until they reach a dangerous level of obesity. Then, because they may begin to feel bad about their physical appearance, they may turn to food to comfort them for their body's negative thoughts and feelings.

This feeling can lead a person to gain weight if these struggles lead to *binge eating*. Binge eating is a disorder that can be seen along with emotional eating much of the time. Binge eating disorder is when a person eats much more than a regular amount of food on a single occasion or sitting, and they feel unable to control themselves or stop themselves. This effect could also be defined as a compulsion to overeat. It has to happen at least two times per week for longer than six months consecutively to be considered a disorder. Binge eating and overeating may appear to be the same, though they are sometimes seen as individual disorders. Overeating is when a person eats more than they require to sustain life. This overeating occurs when they consume much more than they need in a day or a single sitting.

Overeating does not necessarily become binge eating, but it certainly can. Overeating is a general term used to describe the eating disorders that we just defined-Emotional Eating and Binge Eating. Thus, overeating could involve binge eating, food addiction, or other food-related disorders.

Throughout the rest of this book, we will be examining ways to combat this (including using hypnosis) to restore both physical health and a positive mental state to ultimately break the cycle of emotional eating and help you lose weight for good!

The Secret to Lasting Weight Loss

Recognizing the food-related struggles you face will also help you to have a better relationship with your body. Instead of seeing it as; something that you dislike the shape of, something that causes you to feel hungry when you do not need to eat, something that makes you feel guilty when you eat, and something that has disordered eating processes, you can begin to love and care for your body by providing it with nourishment, clean energy, and adequate hydration.

Viewing your body as something to care for (as it is the thing that carries you around all day and houses your most important parts) will allow you to shift your view of yourself and your body to begin seeing it in a more positive light. You can begin to see your body as something you can work together with instead of something you work against.

Recognizing your struggles will also help you to have a better relationship with your mind. Understanding how your mind works will help you to better take care of it. You will be able to recognize your feelings and what they could be caused by, and then treat them in a way that will help it to feel better. Bettering your relationship with food and your body will also improve your relationship with your mind. This relationship will improve because you will begin to feed it what it needs, which will, in turn, lead to better cognitive functioning, control over impulses (like impulses to give in to cravings), and decision-making. This effect will help overall in your relationships with your food, your body, and your mind.

As you can see, dealing with the mind and its struggles is the secret to lasting weight loss and happy life overall. Throughout this book, we will address the mental struggles and help you to break free from them. It will not be an easy process, but it will be well worth it.

Be gentle with yourself throughout this process, as it will be uncomfortable at times and will require strength. This book will help you through it, as you are not alone. I hope that this book also reminds you that many other people are suffering from the same type of food-related disorders as you are and that you are not alone in that either. This book will take a step-by-step approach, which will make for the highest chance of recovery. If at any time you need to take a break to think about the information you have learned, feel free to do so, but make sure you come back to this book quite soon after. Going through this recovery process can be a lot, but it will be possible with the right support.

You have already taken the first step in recovery, which is acknowledging that you have an issue. For that, I congratulate you!

Chapter 2: Emotional Eating

Before we begin looking at the concrete methods that you can use to begin losing weight and breaking free from your mental struggles, we will learn a little more about something called *emotional eating*. I briefly touched on this in the previous chapter, but here we will delve deeper into it before moving on.

What Is Emotional Eating?

As we discussed in the previous chapter, emotional eating occurs when a person suffering from emotional deficiencies of some sort (including a lack of affection, lack of connection, stress, depression, anxiety, or feelings like sadness and anger) eats as a means of gaining comfort from the food they are eating.

Many people find comfort in food. When people experience negative feelings and turn to food consumption to reduce their pain or feel better, this is called emotional eating. Some people do this on occasion, like after a breakup or after a bad fight, but when this occurs at least a few times a week, it negatively impacts one's life. At this point, it becomes an issue that needs to be addressed. Thank you for taking the time to work on yourself in this way, and I am here with you at each step.

What Is Binge Eating?

Another form of disordered eating that is often seen, along with emotional eating, is *binge eating*. I defined this term in the previous chapter, but we will revisit it here briefly.

Binge eating disorder is when a person eats much more than a regular amount of food on a single occasion or sitting, and they feel unable to control themselves or stop themselves. This person could also be experiencing a compulsion to overeat.

To be considered a "Binge Eating Disorder," it must happen at least two times per week for longer than six months consecutively. If this is not the case, it can still negatively affect a person's life, but it would not be considered a Binge Eating Disorder diagnosis.

Why Does Emotional Eating Happen?

Emotional eating occurs because eating foods that we enjoy makes us feel rewarded on our brains' emotional and physiological levels.

People binge eat for a very similar reason to the reason why people experience emotional eating. This reason is that eating foods that we enjoy in terms of taste, smell, texture, etc., makes us feel rewarded on our brains' emotional and physiological level.

Throughout this chapter, we will look more in-depth at these eating disorders to give you more information about why they occur and what could cause them.

How to Tell if You Are Emotionally Eating

Because scientists and psychiatrists understand the brain's chemical reward process when a person emotionally eats, they know that there are different types of food cravings. There are food cravings that indicate emotional deficiencies and the types of cravings that pregnant women experience. Because they understand the science behind it, researchers have come up with ways to tell if some type of emotional deficiency causes a craving.

This method begins by determining the foods that a person craves and when they crave them. For example, if every time someone has a stressful situation, they feel like eating a pizza, or if a person who is depressed tends to eat a lot of chocolate, this could indicate emotional eating. As you know by now, emotional eating and bulimia are closely related, and emotional eating can lead to bulimia over time.

If you crave fruit like a watermelon on a hot day, you are likely just dehydrated, and your body is trying to get water from a water-filled fruit that it knows will make it more hydrated. Examining situations like this has led scientists and psychiatrists to explore eating disorders in more depth and determine what types of emotional deficiencies can manifest themselves through food cravings or disordered eating in this way.

Recognizing your triggers is important because this will allow you to notice when you may be feeling emotional hunger and when you are feeling actual hunger. If you become hungry, you can look back on your day or the last hour and determine if any of your triggers were present. If they were, you would determine that you are likely experiencing emotional hunger, and you can take the appropriate steps instead of giving in to the cravings blindly.

There are many different emotional causes for the cravings we experience. There may be others than those listed in the previous chapter, and these are all valid. A person's emotional eating experience is unique and personal and could be caused by many things. You may also experience a combination of emotional deficiencies or one of those listed in addition to others. Many of these can overlap, such as anxiety and depression, often seen together in a single person. The level of these emotional deficiencies that you experience could indicate the level of emotional eating you struggle with. Whatever experiences or struggles you are dealing with, there is the hope of recovery, and this is what the rest of this book will focus on.

In the next chapter, we will learn several ways to determine your mental state so that you can begin to combat emotional eating.

How to Read Your Hunger

Now that you understand emotional eating, we will look at the different types of hunger and how you can tell them apart. This section will help you distinguish when you are hungry and when you may turn to food to soothe your emotional state.

Real hunger is when our body needs nutrients or energy and lets us know that we should soon replenish our energy. This feeling happens when it has been a few hours since our last meal when we wake up in the morning, or after a lot of strenuous activity like a long hike. Our body uses hunger to signal to us that it needs more energy and that if it doesn't get it soon, it will begin to use our stored energy as fuel. While there is nothing wrong with our body using its stored fuel, it can be used as a sign that we should eat shortly to replenish these stores.

Perceived hunger is when we think we are hungry, but our body doesn't require any more energy or the stores to be replenished. This kind of hunger can happen for several reasons, including an emotional deficiency, a negative mental state, or the occurrence of a psychological trigger.

The Science of Cravings and Food Addictions

We may often see ingredients on the packages of foods we eat, but we aren't sure of exactly what they are, just that they taste good. This section will take a deeper look at them and what they do to your brain.

Casein is a heavily processed ingredient that is derived from milk. It is processed a few times over and eventually creates concentrated milk solids. These milk solids- called Casein are then added into foods like cheese, french fries, milkshakes, and other fast and convenient packaged or fast-foods that contain dairy or dairy products (such as pastries and salad dressings). Casein has been compared to nicotine in its addictive properties. It is often seen in cheese, and this is why there is increasing evidence that people can become, and many are already addicted to cheese. The reason for this is during digestion. When cheese and other foods that contain Casein are digested, it is broken down, and one of the compounds that it breaks down into is a compound that is strikingly similar to opioids. This highly addictive substance is in pain killers.

High fructose corn syrup is surely an ingredient you have heard of before or at least one you have seen on the packaging of your favorite snacks or quick foods. While this is derived from real corn, after it is finished being processed, there is nothing corn-like about it. High fructose corn syrup is essentially the same thing as refined sugar when all is said and done. It is used as a sweetener in foods like soda, cereal, and other sweet and quick foods. This ingredient is often seen because it is much cheaper than using sugar and is much easier to work with.

High Fructose Corn Syrup is another common food additive that is highly addictive. This substance is similar to cocaine in its addictive properties.

MSG stands for Monosodium Glutamate, which sounds a lot like a chemical you may have encountered in science class in college. MSG is added to foods to give them a delicious flavor. It is essentially a very concentrated form of salt. What this does (in foods such as fast-food, packaged convenience foods, and buffet-style food) is that it gives it that wonderfully salty and fatty flavor that makes us keep coming back for more. Companies put this in food because it comes at an extremely low cost, and the flavor it brings covers up the artificial flavors of all of the other cheap ingredients used to make these foods. MSG has been known to block our natural appetite suppressant, which normally kicks in when we have had enough to eat. For this reason, when we are eating foods containing MSG, we do not recognize when we are satiated, and we continue to eat until we are stuffed because it tastes so great.

Sugar Addictions: The Real Devil

We will now look more closely at sugar and how it affects our bodies and our minds. Sugar is the worst culprit of all of these food additives. Sugar is responsible for this because it is so hard to avoid! Sugar is found in everything we eat that we can buy from a restaurant or a store. There are many sugar forms and so many names disguised as in the ingredients list on food packaging. One food may contain 70 percent sugar, but on the label, it may look as if this is not true because the different types of sugar have all been separated to trick us into thinking this is not the case. When it comes to avoiding sugar, it takes diligence and a keen eye for detail.

We already discussed one form of sugar, High Fructose Corn Syrup. This sugar type is cheap and easy to get your hands on, so it is added to virtually everything packaged that we can ingest. It is added because it gives even salty foods that tasty flavor balance.

As we discussed previously in this chapter, the chemicals found in food act in our brains very similar to how highly addictive drugs act. Sugar itself acts in a specific way that makes it so difficult to avoid. Sugar affects what is called the *Limbic System*. The limbic system is a group of structures in the brain that have to do with our emotions and memory. This system includes the regulation of our emotions and forming memories, which contributes to our learning.

For this reason, when we eat something very sugary, the chemicals that make up the sugars can affect our emotions. When this happens, it makes us feel emotions like happiness and satisfaction. Then, because eating certain foods makes us feel like this, we form a memory of this, and in turn, we learn that eating these specific foods gives us positive emotions. These emotions make us keep coming back for more.

So, when we eat something that contains both sugars and Casein, for example, we will get action on our limbic system and our reward system in the brain. Therefore, foods that give us both a feeling of reward and a surge of positive emotion are the most difficult to resist and the first ones we turn to when we want comfort in the form of food because we know they will make us feel good. And they always do, as these chemical reactions in the brain occur each time. We may not even realize this, as it becomes second nature to us. We may not recognize the positive feelings we get after we eat something that comforts us, but we know we keep craving it for some reason. If this has ever happened to you, you now know why this is. After learning about these things, pay attention to your cravings and see if this may be the explanation for why you have them. Pay attention also to the times that these cravings occur. Did you just receive some bad news? Was it on a rainy day when you were feeling especially down? Hold onto this information as we will revisit it shortly. Later on, in this book, we will also be discussing several ways to overcome these challenges to break the cycles of emotional eating and overeating.

How to Change Your Relationship With Food

The key to solving the food-related struggles that you face is to address your core wounds. Understanding how your mind works will help you to better take care of it. You will be able to recognize your feelings and how they could have come about, and then treat them in a way that will help it to feel better. Bettering your relationship with food and your body will also improve your relationship with your mind. This relationship will then allow you to begin to feed it what it needs, which will, in turn, lead to better cognitive functioning, control over impulses, and decision-making. This better functioning will help overall your relationship with your food, body, and mind.

In the next chapter, we will take a deeper look into these core wounds, and I will begin teaching you strategies to deal with them. Through the next chapter and those that follow, we will begin learning how to deal with emotional eating.

Chapter 3: Addressing Your Current Mental State

In this chapter, we will look at how you can begin to tackle your mind to make positive changes for your body and break free from your eating disorder once and for all.

We will begin by looking at core wounds before learning how to deal with them and ultimately change your relationship with food.

What Are Core Wounds?

As discussed in the previous chapter, there are several types of emotional deficiencies indicated by disordered eating. Once you have determined which of these emotional deficiencies (or which combination of them) are present in your life, you can begin to look at them in a little more detail. By doing so, you will come upon your core wounds. A core wound is something that you believe to be true about yourself or your life, and it is something that likely came about as a result of a coping mechanism you developed to deal with childhood. For example, this could be something like; the feeling of not being enough, the belief that you are unlovable, or the belief that you are stupid.

How to Address Your Core Wounds

By understanding and addressing your core wounds, you will be able to change your behaviors because of the intricate relationship that exists between your thoughts, your emotions, and your behaviors. By addressing your thoughts and emotions, you will change your behaviors and free yourself from eating disordered. You may be wondering how you can begin to address your core wounds, as it can be difficult to know where to begin.

The first step is learning to control and change your thoughts, which, in turn, leads to changes in your behavior. By taking control of your thoughts and beliefs, they don't have the opportunity to manifest into unhealthy behaviors such as overeating, turning to food for comfort, or any other unhealthy coping mechanisms that you have developed throughout your life.

Becoming aware of your thoughts is the most crucial step in this entire guide, as everything else will fail without it. Paying attention to your thoughts will help you identify what thoughts are going through your mind during an intense emotional moment. By looking deep within, to get in touch with your deepest feelings, you will be more likely to succeed in weight loss and overall lifestyle improvement.

Journaling

One great example of how to put this into practice is through the use of journaling. Journaling can help in a process such as this because it can help you organize your thoughts and feelings and visually see what is working and what isn't working for you. While we can give tips and examples, every person is different, so to find exactly what works for you, you will have to try different things and see which techniques help you personally the most and in the best way. Journaling can be about anything like how you feel since beginning a new program, how you feel physically since changing your diet, how you feel emotionally now that you are not reaching for food to comfort your emotions and anything along these lines.

Self-Reflection

Doing some serious and deep self-reflection is not an easy process but a necessary one for healing yourself and changing your habits that are so ingrained. Looking deep within and asking yourself the proper questions will help you take the first step, acknowledging the issues and finding their sources. Finding the sources will tell you exactly what you need to face and deal with to achieve a lasting change of this new intuitive eating lifestyle.

If changing your life is a distraction from the underlying issues, the change will not be lasting. These issues will rise to the surface again eventually, and they will manifest themselves in strong cravings. I want you to permanently change your life, and to do this; we will begin with some deep self-reflection. You will get out of this workbook what you put in, so take your time as you go through this chapter and try to get in touch with the deeper parts of yourself.

We will begin the self-reflection with some questions to ask yourself to get into a self-examination mindset. Complete this workbook, and you will be well on your way to dealing with your emotions, as you will have a better idea of what these emotions are.

1. Do I feel like I struggle with emotional eating?

Yes ____ No ____

2. Do I wish to find out the underlying causes of my emotional eating?

Yes ____ No ____

3. Do I feel like it is time for a lifestyle change in terms of my eating habits?

Yes ____ No ____

The first question you will ask yourself is a rather obvious one, but this will make it easy for you to get a start on your self-examination.

1. Have I been diagnosed with mood-related disorders (such as depression, bipolar disorder, or anxiety)?

Yes ____ No____

If your answer is yes, you skip section 2. If you answered No and you are unsure if you suffer from one of these, complete section 2.

2. Do I have long periods of low mood or an anxious state?

Yes ____ No ____

3. Have I been feeling this way for the last 3 to 6 months?

Yes ____ No ____

4. Do I often feel disconnected from my life?

Yes ____ No ____

5. Do I often feel nervous and worried about worst-case scenarios?

Yes ____ No ____

6. Do I often catastrophize in my head when thinking about things that are to come?

Yes ____ No ____

7. Do I often feel drastic swings between very high moods (like happy, excited, and motivated) and very low moods (sad, down, hopeless)

Yes ____ No ____

If you answered mostly Yes to the questions above, you might suffer from a mood-related disorder. While this questionnaire is not conclusive and is not sanctioned by a doctor or a medical professional, this could give you a bit of direction regarding your mood, emotions, and the causes of your emotional eating. Knowing that the cause could be something like depression, anxiety, or another mood disorder can give you some clarity on your mental state. If you think this could be the case, consider visiting your doctor to discuss this further with someone who is especially knowledgeable in these areas.

Acknowledging Your Emotions

It is very important to notice and address your feelings, as they can tell you many important things.

Pay attention to your thoughts, and whenever you feel a negative emotion, work backward. Try to figure out what thoughts were just on your mind before you felt negative emotions. Emotions that you should be looking out for are stress, anxiety, self-loathing, sadness, demotivation, anger, and frustration. These emotions are the ones that typically cause a person to choose instant gratification.

Just like how you will be paying attention to the thoughts that occurred before feeling a negative emotion, pay attention to the thoughts that occurred before feeling a positive emotion. By identifying what those thoughts were, you will begin to learn what types of thoughts bring positive emotions. Typically, when a person feels positive emotions, it creates more motivation and inspiration to reach goals.

One great way to begin feeling your emotions is by self-reflecting and noticing when they are causing you struggles related to food. Below are some more specific questions that will help prompt you to look at your emotions more deeply.

- Emotional Triggers

What are some triggers related to your emotions or specific emotions that make you seek comfort in the form of food? For example: When I feel scared, I begin to crave sweets.

- Additional Triggers

Are there any other triggers that you experience that cause your emotional deficiencies to flare up? For example: When I go to school, I feel lonely.

Recognizing your triggers is important because this will allow you to notice when you may be feeling emotional hunger and when you are feeling actual hunger. If you become hungry, you can look back on your day or the last hour and determine if any of your triggers were present. If they were, you would be able to determine that you are likely experiencing emotional hunger, and you can take the appropriate steps instead of giving in to the cravings blindly. These triggers tie into emotional eating because when you experience a trigger that causes one of your emotional deficiencies to become more apparent to you (or to act up), you are most likely to turn to food as a means of comfort and as a way to self-soothe. Recognizing what these triggers are will help you to recognize when to intervene in your normal cognitive processes such as "I am hungry" "I am going to eat a cookie." Instead of this normal process that would occur after a situation or an emotion triggers your feelings of loneliness, for example, you will know to intervene, and instead, it will go something like this; "I am hungry," "Am I hungry or feeling an emotional need?", "A trigger just occurred, so I am going to call a friend and talk instead of eating what I crave."

Using Positive Self-Talk

Once you have addressed your emotions and your core wounds, you can begin to intervene and change them to result in healthier behaviors. You will do this using positive self-talk. Adopting helpful thought processes fosters better emotions overall, which leads to more productive behaviors.

When people have developed unhelpful thinking processes, it is hard to make decisions that will benefit their future selves because their thoughts create negative emotions that drive away motivation. This situation is where something called *positive self-talk* can come in. Positive self-talk can be instrumental in helping you to recover from disordered eating.

What Is Positive Self-Talk?

Their inner critic controls many people's minds. The inner critic shares words with you, such as "You should just give up" Or "What makes you think you'll succeed?" which is rooted in the opposite of positive self-talk- Negative self-talk!

Instead of creating an open space that allows for mistakes, growth, and development, your inner critic causes you to question your worth. This questioning makes it difficult for you to have the positive, growth mindset needed to complete tasks and go after things that may be difficult to achieve. In this case, helping your mind begin using positive self-talk will help you recover for the long-term.

How Can You Begin Using Positive Self-Talk?

Below are several ways that you can begin to use positive self-talk. Over time, your mind will get used to thinking in this way, and you will find it much easier to do.

1. Remind yourself

Bad habits are built through many years, and no amount of willpower can undo a lifetime of bad habits, such as a strong inner critic that uses negative self-talk. By rewiring your brain to minimize the amount of negativity you feel in the first place, you will eventually get used to filling your mind with positive thoughts instead of negative ones.

2. Stop the automatic process of negativity.

Often, if the person had just paid attention to their thought process, they would be able to catch themselves before their mind automatically spiraled to a place of complete demotivation. By catching yourself before you get there, you can prevent yourself from falling into your negative thought patterns, limiting you and holding you back.

3. Find positive influences

Surrounding yourself with people that can encourage you and foster positivity will also change your inner-critic's opinion. Often, hearing positive compliments from other people hold a heavier weight in the eyes of your inner-critic compared to you telling your inner-critic the same thing. Try spending time with people who support your goals and the changes you are looking to make in your life. It will make your journey a little bit easier.

4. Limit Negative Influences

By limiting your life's negative influences, you are making a statement to yourself that you place importance on preserving your mental health. When you remove negative influences and limit your exposure to things or people that make you feel negative, you prioritize yourself, which is a great way to practice self-care.

5. Practice a gratitude exercise

This exercise is a great exercise to remind yourself of everything you love and appreciate yourself and your life. Take time to write down all of the things that you love about yourself and your life. Doing this will remind you of all of the positivity surrounding you and will serve to uplift you.

Chapter 4: More Ways to Challenge Your Mind

In this chapter, we will look at how you can begin to tackle your mind to make positive changes for your body and break free from your eating disorder once and for all.

How Self-Care Can Help

Self-Care is the method by which you will begin to love and to take care of your body. Self-care includes both your physical and your mental health. When you begin to take care of yourself physically and mentally, you will begin to see many changes come about, namely an increase in positive feelings and a decrease in negative ones.

How to Practice Self-Care

There are numerous ways that you can practice self-care, and these ways can be different for everyone. In this section, I will outline some ways to practice self-care to begin feeling more positive about yourself and your body and begin changing your internal environment around you.

- You Are Worthy

This exercise is a great exercise to remind yourself of everything you love and appreciate yourself and your life. Take time to write down all of the things that you love about yourself and your life. Doing this will remind you of all of the positivity surrounding you and will serve to uplift you.

- Limit Negative Influences

By limiting your life's negative influences, you are making a statement to yourself that you place importance on preserving your mental health. When you remove negative influences and limit your exposure to things or people that make you feel negative, you prioritize yourself, which is a great way to practice self-care.

Included here are also the negative influences that you have over yourself. Limiting beliefs and negative self-talk, and a negative body image can lead a person to feel terrible about themselves, often to the point of feeling like they hate themselves. As I mentioned earlier, to make lasting changes, we will work on loving ourselves instead of hating ourselves. By positively seeing your body, you will begin to make choices with your body's health in mind because of all of the things it allows you to do. This process will lead to lasting, positive changes for your physical and mental health.

- Support System

Finding a positive and uplifting support system helps improve and preserve your mental health. This system can be one person or a group of people. It can include family or friends or acquaintances, as long as they support you in your journey and help you to feel positive about your life and yourself in general. Some examples of places you can find a support system include Facebook groups, support groups, weight loss support groups, and books. Not only will a support system help you to move toward positivity, but when you begin to make changes in your life, your support system will help by supporting you in maintaining these changes.

- Journaling

Another journaling exercise you can do to change your limiting beliefs is writing down all of the limiting beliefs you think you possess. Then, try to think of and write down where you think they came from. For example, try to think of where you learned to think this way or where this was modeled for you. Having this information written down in front of you can help you to begin changing them, as awareness is the first step to change.

- Notice And Challenge Your Inner Critic

The negative self-talk that many people experience comes from something called their *inner critic*. Your inner critic lives in a black and white world, a world with very little room for the grey area, and where failure is the worst possible outcome of every scenario. Your inner critic shares words with you, such as, "You should just give up" Or "What makes you think you'll succeed?" Instead of creating an open space that allows for mistakes, growth, and development, your inner critic causes you to question your worth. These thoughts make it difficult for you to have the positive, growth mindset needed to complete tasks and go after things that may be difficult to achieve. For some people, their inner critic is reminiscent of a voice from their past- it could be their mother, father, or person who bullied them. For others, it could simply be their voice criticizing them for everything they do. Sometimes, if a person makes an offhand comment at you, this could lead you to absorb it so deeply that the words they said become a part of your identity.

Awareness is the first step that needs to be taken to recognize your inner-critic and reshape it into something less critical and more supportive. Try to pay attention the next time you are feeling distracted, numb, or anxious. Try to identify whose voice is the voice of your inner critic. Try to find the situation where your inner critic awakens. Allows yourself to dig deep and identify the most vulnerable feelings during situations where your inner critic is awake. These feelings or these situations are likely what your inner critic is trying to protect you from feeling. However, by protecting you, they are holding you back from meeting your full potential.

Using Meditation

Simply put, meditation is a practice where a person uses a technique, like mindfulness - to focus their thoughts and mind on an activity, thought, or object to train their awareness and attention. The goal of this is to help the person achieve clear-headedness and an emotionally calm and stable state.

The simplest methods of meditation all surround achieving mindfulness. Achieving mindfulness is the most popular goal for meditators as it increases overall life satisfaction. Life satisfaction increases when you decrease stress, anxiety, and insomnia. Throughout this book, you will find tips and guides on how to combat psychological challenges. You will learn the simplest form of meditation to incorporating meditation in all your day to day activities. You will begin to understand how meditation will help you begin learning to love yourself and let go of negative thoughts. You will learn how to achieve a non-judgmental state of mind that will free your mind to accept everybody.

Related to meditation is something called *visualization*. Visualization is a type of inner transformation that leads to seeing actual results in reality. Visualization is also a form of creative thinking where people can shape their lives using a specific purpose within their minds. The best part about the image is that a person may have envisioned that it doesn't have to rely upon the outer world's external events. It can depend entirely on a person's imagination and the act of manifesting certain things. This idea will become relevant in the next section when we begin practicing meditation.

Meditation Techniques

In this ten-step guide, we will be using a mix of visualization and meditation to guide you into focusing on your goals. This guide is very similar to what we learned with visualization; researchers have found that visualizing and meditating on the process of a person achieving their goals will help them to do it in real life. Try these following steps of guided meditation to help put your goal into the future:

1. Start by thinking of an area of your life in your mind. Choose something where you

have been struggling with, or you would like to change.
2. Now start to imagine the best possible outcome you would like to live in concerning the area you've selected. Imagine these 6 to 12 months from now. What is the reality that you are looking to achieve? Try not to get caught up with any negativity or limitations; instead, just allow yourself to imagine and get carried away with your strongest goals.
3. Focus your mind on connecting with just one goal you would like to achieve over the next three months. Make sure your goal is a good one and is as meaningful as possible. If you choose a goal that is not meaningful or doesn't hold a lot of weight, the result won't feel special for you. Make sure to choose something significant enough to feel a high sense of accomplishment and motivation for your next goal once you achieve this goal. Be sure to run your goal through the SMART acronym to ensure that it is a goal that is set up for success.
4. Now that you are starting to feel connected with the goal that you've set, try to imagine what your life will be like once you achieve the goal. Visualize a picture or movie and try to view it as if you are looking at it through your pair of eyes. Factor in all the other sensory perceptions to try to imagine the most real and positive feelings. Where are you? Who is with you? What are the things happening around you?

5. Now, begin to step out of that picture or movie you've imagined and begin to imagine yourself floating up in the air where you are sitting now while taking that imagery with you. Take a deep breath and as you breathe out, use your breath to give life to the image and fill it with intention and positive energy. Repeat this five times.
6. In this step, it is time to imagine yourself floating out into the future while imagining yourself dropping the imagery you've created for your goal down into your real-life below you at the exact time and date you've set for yourself to reach this goal.
7. Pay attention to the things that need to happen between then and now and how it is beginning to re-evaluate itself to support you in achieving that goal. Visualize this process and all those events to make it feel as realistic as possible.
8. Once you feel like that step is complete, bring your awareness back to the present, and with your eyes still shut, start to think about what steps you will need to take in the next few days that will help you move closer to achieving your goal.
9. Take a few more deep breaths to ground yourself to the present before opening your eyes. Before you forget, write down a list of steps that you need to take to achieve your goal or begin to write down your experience in your journal, so you don't forget.
10. In this last step, you will focus on taking action and staying focused. Make sure that

you are doing something that brings you closer to achieving your goal daily.

Use this meditation and visualization technique once a week after you first complete the steps. Doing this once a week helps you continue to move forward towards your end goal and help you bring your vision into real life. Seeing is believing, so using your mind and meditation can create the best future that you have imagined for yourself.

What Is Mindful Eating?

There are many activities in your life that you may not even think that meditation can impact. In this section, we will discuss how incorporating meditation techniques into the act of eating will help you change your relationship with food and develop healthier rituals around eating. This technique is called *mindful eating*. Mindful eating is a technique that is done which incorporates mindfulness with eating. This technique helps people combat common food-related disorders, including emotional eating and binge eating that are so prevalent in our fast-paced lives.

Mindful eating is important because eating is one of the tasks that we perform numerous times every day of our lives. When we do a certain task repeatedly, our bodies will naturally try to automate that action to save us energy. However, when we eat mindlessly, we don't pay attention to the way food tastes, what we're eating, and how quickly we consume it. This automation causes people to mistreat their bodies without knowing. Fear not, as I will teach you how to begin using mindful eating to your benefit and provide you with some exercises to help you begin incorporating this into your daily life.

The Benefits Of Mindful Eating

Forgetting to eat mindfully is something that most of our population struggles with, and they don't even know it. This struggle happens because our lives function at such a fast pace that we don't put much thought into the details surrounding the act of eating.

We typically find ourselves eating at work, in front of our computer, eating dinner in front of the TV, or eating during the commute to work! This seemingly insignificant detail is one of the leading factors contributing to today's obesity and eating disorder problem. To combat this, we need to improve our relationship with eating and our eating rituals. This improvement comes down to an ability to eat mindfully.

Overall, practicing mindful eating will enhance your enjoyment of meals, prevent overeating, help with digestion, reduce anxiety about food-related matters, and better the relationship that you have with eating and food.

When and How to Use Mindful Eating

The goal of mindful eating is to shift your mind's focus from external thoughts to thoughts of exploration and enjoyment of the eating experience itself. We do this to develop a new mindset around food and a new relationship with food and the act of eating.

Here are a couple of points to come back to that will help you identify when you are eating mindlessly and switch to a mindful eating form.

1. You are consistently eating until the point of being full or even feeling physically il
2. You tend to nibble on snacks but don't taste them
3. You aren't don't notice what you eat, and you often find yourself eating meals in places that surround you with distractions
4. You are rushing through your meals
5. You have trouble remembering what you ate, or even the taste and smell of the last meal you've consumed

If you find yourself relating to any or all of the points that I just mentioned, you will surely benefit from mindful eating.

The Mindful Eating Technique

I will now share the technique of mindful eating with you. Next time you sit down for a meal, follow these tips to practice mindful eating and try to make it a daily habit.

1. Prioritize your mealtimes. Try to isolate a 15-minute block to take a seat and savour your food.

2. Be sure to get rid of any distractions present while you eat. You cannot enjoy the food you eat when you are not focused on it. Try asking yourself how often you eat sitting in front of the TV, in the car, or in front of the computer? Under those circumstances, eating is always mindless which can make you overeat, choose unhealthy foods for yourself, or neglecting to enjoy the food you are eating.
3. Try not to rush during meal times. Plan a time block in which you will eat, and make sure that you don't have any distractions around you. Even eating with a coworker or a friend may be a distraction due to conversation.
4. Always sit down to eat your meal. Try and avoid eating while standing up or walking as these create distractions.
5. Serve your meal on a plate or bowl. If possible, serve it on your favorite plate or bowl. Avoid eating food from the packet or take out containers as it makes eating feel less formal.
6. Ensure that you chew each bite thoroughly. Many people find themselves swallowing too soon and end up with digestion problems. Give your stomach an easier time digesting by breaking down the food properly before swallowing.
7. Make sure to only eat until you're 80% full. This level is a fine line. Don't eat until you are certain you are full, but eat until you feel satisfied. A lot of the time, the feeling of

fullness comes 10 minutes after you finish your meal. If you find yourself feeling full while you are still eating, you probably have overeaten.
8. Take your time to truly savor the taste of food. Use all five of your senses. Before eating, take a look at your meal of its look, smell, and overall appeal. Think about how each ingredient was cooked and seasoned and how you think the dish would taste because of it. During the meal, identify the taste of all the ingredients. What is the flavor? How does the flavor change if I eat different combinations of the ingredients? What does it smell like? What does the texture feel like on your tongue?
9. Think about how the meal is making you feel. Is it happy? Pleasurable? Guilty? Regretful? Stressed out? Disappointed? Pay attention to the thoughts that the food leads you to think. Do you think about specific memories? Fearful thoughts? Beliefs about anything? How does your body feel after the meal compared to before? Do you feel energetic after the meal, or does it make you tired? Is your stomach empty or full?
10. Try to make meals for yourself instead of buying them, when possible. The act of preparing food is proven to be psychologically beneficial and therapeutic. Make sure you are touching, tasting, and smelling the individual ingredients.
11. Make a note of the difference in good food. This difference tends to be food that is fresh,

seasonal, and minimally processed. Fresh and organic food tends to improve your overall mood and health. Food is our body's nourishment, and it provides the nutrition necessary for us to function optimally. Ingesting better quality food and ingredients is crucial to helping you feel better physically and psychologically.

Practicing meditation is your first step in being able to achieve mindful eating. Allowing yourself to be mindful in your day-to-day life will bring new joys and satisfactions that have always been there but have not been noticed in some time.

Chapter 5: Food-Related Changes to Begin Making

This chapter will provide you with a solid foundation of knowledge on which to build your new lifestyle. We will look at how intuitive eating can answer all of your struggles and help you find recovery.

Making Good Food-Related Choices

As we discussed earlier in this book, making good choices begins with self-exploration and a deep look into your core wounds. Once you have done this, you can begin to make positive decisions for your health and life, and over time these will become more and more habitual. We will spend this chapter looking at some of how you can begin to make good choices related to food and eating.

How to Begin Making Good Choices Using Intuitive Eating

One great way to make good choices when it comes to food is by using something called intuitive eating. Below, I will define intuitive eating for you and give you insight into how this can change your life.

What Is Intuitive Eating?

Intuitive eating is a new perspective from which to view how you feed your body. This eating style puts you in control. Instead of following a list of pre-

designed guidelines about when and what to eat. Intuitive eating encourages you to listen to your body and listen to the signals it sends you regarding;
- what to eat
- how much to eat
- when to eat.

Paying attention to these signals ensures that you are giving your body exactly what it needs when it needs it, instead of forcing it into a specific kind of diet.

Intuitive eating does not limit any specific foods and does not require you to exclusively stick to certain foods. Instead, it encourages you to learn as much as you can about what your body is telling you and follow its signals.

The two main components of the intuitive eating philosophy are eating when you are hungry and stopping eating when you are satiated. This concept may seem like a no-brainer, but we are very far from eating intuitively, as odd as it may seem in today's societies. With so many diet trends and numerous "rules" for how you should and should not eat, it can be difficult to put these ideas aside and let your body guide you exclusively.

The philosophy behind intuitive eating is that if you wait until you are too hungry before eating, you will be much more likely to overeat or binge eat. You should do this because, by this time, you be feeling ravenous instead of mildly hungry. If, instead, you choose to adhere to your hunger and eat when your body tells you that it needs sustenance, you will be much more likely to eat just the right amount. As a result, your body will be satisfied rather than completely stuffed, and instead of feeling shameful and angry that you have eaten, you can feel happy that you have provided your body with what it needed. This act requires you to listen to and respect what your body is telling you and then provide it with nutrients to keep working hard for you!

The Benefits of Intuitive Eating

One of the reasons that intuitive eating is such a successful and cherished form of eating is that it allows the body to lead the mind in the right direction when seeking out its needs. Below, we will look at the benefits of letting your body guide your eating choices.

- Allows the body to get what it needs

Did you know that your cravings could be giving you much more information than you give them credit for?

A craving is an intense longing for something (in this case food), that comes about intensely and feels urgent. In our case, that longing is for s a very specific type of food. When we have cravings for certain foods, it can mean more than what it seems.

While you may think that craving is an indication of hunger or a desire for the taste of a certain food, it may indicate that your body is low on certain vitamins or minerals. As a result, your body seeks out a certain food that it thinks will provide it with this vitamin or mineral. This requirement reaches your consciousness in the form of an intense craving. In this case, the body is trying to help itself by telling you what to eat. For this reason, understanding your cravings could help you give your body exactly what it is longing for.

For example, if you are craving juice or pop or other sugary drinks like this, consider that you might, in fact, be dehydrated and, therefore, thirsty. Sometimes we see drinks in our fridge, and since we are thirsty, we want them. Next time you are craving a sugary drink, try having a glass of water first, then wait a few minutes and see if you are still craving that Coca-Cola. You may not want it anymore once your thirst is quenched.

If you are craving meat, you may feel like you want some fried chicken or a hot dog. This craving could indicate a deficit of iron or protein. The best protein sources are chicken breast cooked in the oven, and iron is best received from spinach, oysters, or lentils. If you think you may not like these foods, there are many different ways to prepare them, and you can likely find a way you like.

- Prevents overeating

It can be hard to know how much to eat and when you have had enough to eat without letting yourself eat too much. Sometimes people will eat until the point that they begin to feel full. Often, we keep eating until we become stuffed, even to the point of making ourselves feel physically ill. Intuitive eating will help you avoid this, as this kind of eating encourages you to give your body what it needs to take great care of it. Stuffing your body until it is too full is not what your body is asking for, and once you become accustomed to listening to your body's needs, you will know when it is time to stop.

- Helps you break free from self-judgment

Intuitive eating will help you to finally make peace with your body and yourself as a whole. It does this by showing you that your body has needs and that there is no shame intending to these needs, as long as you do so in a healthy way.

You cannot fully embrace and practice intuitive eating if you have those nagging feelings of self-judgment each time you take a bite of food or decide that you will eat lunch when you are hungry. For this reason, to practice intuitive eating, you must understand that feeding your body is an act of compassion for yourself and that this does not need to come with self-judgment.

- It is inclusive, not exclusive.

One of the great things about this eating style is that it is not founded on restricting a person's intake of certain foods or allowing only a small variety of foods.

Diets like this are extremely hard to transition to and are hard to maintain for a long period. Intuitive eating is about including as many natural whole foods as you wish while also ensuring that you consume enough of your nutrients. With this style of eating, you can eat whatever you wish, whenever you wish. This part makes it much easier to stick with this type of diet and reduces the chances of falling off after a short period due to cravings or intense hunger. It does not restrict calories or reduce your intake greatly, making it easier to handle than a traditional diet for many people. It feels natural to eat in this way, which makes it effective.

How to Make Intuitive Eating Part of Your Life

One of the best ways to make this type of eating a part of your life is to practice it with intention. This intention is especially important when you are just beginning. Each time you feel a pang of hunger or a compulsion to eat, take a minute to examine your inner world. By doing this, you will get your mind and body accustomed to working together. Also, do the same after you eat. By doing these two things, you will ensure that you are eating when hungry and stopping when satisfied.

When you finish eating a meal, rank your fullness level on a scale of 1 to 10, 1 being extremely hungry and ten being extremely stuffed. This ranking will help you determine if you are successfully stopping when you are satisfied and not overeating.

It is also important that you learn how to deal with your emotions and feelings effectively without using food. Using the techniques you have learned in this book, you will address your inner demons, making space for you to listen to your body and its needs.

As you know by now, listening to your body, your emotions, and your mind is extremely important when it comes to practicing intuitive eating. As long as you remember this, you will be well on your way to becoming a lifelong intuitive eater.

What Kind of Foods Should You Choose?

Fish is a great way to get healthy fats into your diet. Certain fish are very low in carbohydrates but high in good fats, making them perfect for a healthy diet. They also contain minerals and vitamins that will be good for your health. Salmon is a great fish to eat, as it is versatile and delicious. Many fish also include essential fatty acids that we can only get through our diet. Other fish that are good for you include:
- Sardines
- Mackerel
- Herring
- Trout
- Albacore Tuna

Meat and Poultry make up a large part of most Americans' diets. Meats and Poultry that are fresh and not processed do not include any carbohydrates and contain high protein levels. Eating lean meats helps to maintain your strength and muscle mass and gives you energy for hours. Grass-fed meats, in particular, are rich in antioxidants.

Eggs are another amazing, protein-filled food. Eggs help your body feel satiated for longer and keep your blood sugar levels consistent, which is great for overall health. The whole egg is good for you, as the yolk is where the nutrients are. The cholesterol found within egg yolks also has been demonstrated to lower your risk of getting diseases like heart diseases, despite what most people think. Therefore, do not be afraid of the egg yolk!

Legumes are a great source of protein and fiber, and there are many different types to choose from. These include the following:
- All sorts of beans, including black beans, green beans, and kidney beans
- Peas
- Lentils of all colors
- Chickpeas
- Peas

Examples of fruits that you can eat include the following:
- Citrus fruits such as oranges, grapefruits, lemons, and limes
- Melons of a variety of sorts
- Apples
- Bananas
- Berries including strawberries, blueberries, blackberries, raspberries, and so on
- Grapes

Vegetables are a great source of energy and nutrients, and they include a wide range of naturally

occurring vivid colors, which should all be included in your diet.
- Carrots
- Broccoli and cauliflower
- Asparagus
- Kale
- All sorts of peppers, including hot peppers, bell peppers
- Tomatoes
- Root vegetables (that are a good source of healthy, complete carbohydrates) such as potatoes, sweet potatoes, all types of squash, and beets.

Seeds are another great source of nutrients, vitamins, and minerals, and they are very versatile. These include the following:
- Sesame seeds
- Pumpkin seeds
- Sunflower seeds
- Hemp, flax, and chia seeds are all especially good for your health

Nuts are a great way to get protein if you choose not to eat meat or vegan. They also are packed with nutrients. Some examples are below.
- Almonds
- Brazil Nuts
- Cashews
- Macadamia nuts
- Pistachios
- Pecans

Some healthy fats are essential components of any person's diet, as our bodies cannot make the beneficial compounds that they contain; thus, we rely solely on our diet to get them. These compounds are Omega-3 Fatty Acids, monounsaturated and polyunsaturated fats. Below are some healthy sources of these compounds:
- Avocados
- Healthy, plant-based oils including olive oil and canola oil
- Hemp, chia, and flax seeds
- Walnuts

When it comes to carbohydrates, these should be consumed in **whole grains**, as they are high in fiber, which will help prevent overeating. Whole grains also include essential minerals- those that we can only get from our diet, just like those essential compounds found in healthy fats. These essential minerals are selenium, magnesium, and copper. Sources of these whole grains include the following:
- Quinoa
- Rye, Barley, buckwheat
- Whole grain oats
- Brown rice
- Whole grain bread can be hard to find these days in the grocery store, as many brown loaves of bread disguise themselves as whole grain when, in fact, they are not. However, there are whole grain loaves of bread if you take the time to look at the ingredients list.

Electrolytes

When you first begin losing weight, having Electrolyte depletion is quite common. This depletion is because of water weight loss through fat, thus reducing electrolytes present in your body. Taking electrolyte supplements can help avoid a deficiency in common electrolytes, like magnesium, potassium, and sodium. This depletion is also why you should ensure you are getting enough dietary sodium, as this is an electrolyte that you need. Along with this, though, you will need to ensure you are drinking enough water to avoid dehydration.

Vitamin D

Vitamin D is found in some foods that have been fortified with it, but it can be found in only a few foods in a natural sense. These include cheese, fatty fish like salmon and tuna, as well as egg yolks. Another source is mushrooms that have been exposed to UV rays, so the organic ones are likely of this sort.

Vitamin D can be absorbed naturally through sun exposure, so if you live in a sunny place, make sure you get out for some walks or some timer with the sun on your skin. If you live in a colder or more gloomy place, consider purchasing a lamp that mimics the sun and provides you with vitamin D in your house. On a sunny day, even if it is cold, going outside and getting sun on your face will give you vitamin D.

Chapter 6: Weight Loss

Weight loss is never an easy task, and having the right mindset is crucial to your success, as we have seen throughout this book. Throughout this chapter, we will learn about weight loss and how best to set yourself up for success in this way!

Weight loss is something many people are chasing in the world today, but many of them are going about it in all of the wrong ways. Below, we will look at how you can achieve weight loss without using diets and how this relates to intuitive eating and exercise.

How to Achieve Weight Loss Without Using Diets

A combination of intuitive eating and exercise is the best way to achieve weight loss without using diets! As you have seen, intuitive eating is the best way to get in touch with your inner self, which this book is all about. Below, we will learn about the science of weight loss to better understand how it works within your body.

By taking control of your thoughts and beliefs, they don't have the opportunity to manifest into unhealthy behaviors such as overeating, turning to food for comfort, or any other unhealthy coping mechanisms that you have developed throughout your life. This concept is a through-line in this book, and it is something that I want you to remember for the rest of your life. You do not need diets to find a healthier you!

The Science of Weight Loss

If you are reading this book to lose weight, you will need to ensure that you understand the science of weight loss. The basic mathematical equation to represent weight loss is the following;

Calories in − (minus) Calories used for basic survival (for example, walking, eating, breathing) - (minus) Calories burned from exercise = (equals)

The number that results from this equation (in the equals position) will either be positive or negative.

- If the number is positive, this means that you ingested more calories than you burned. If the number is positive, you can envision it as having more energy than you could use. When this occurs, the extra energy is stored as fat in the body.
- If the number is negative, this means that you burned more calories than you ingested. If the number is negative, you used more energy than you had, which translates to weight loss. This effect happens because once the readily available energy in your body is all used up, the body's fat storage will begin to be used for additional energy, resulting in a loss of weight in the form of fat.
- If the number is zero, calories ingested and calories burned are equal. If the number is zero, this indicates "breaking even" in terms of your energy.

This equation explains how falling off the diet for one meal or two each day could lead to the maintenance of the same weight or even an increase in weight in some cases. This equation also shows us that weight gain or weight loss comes down to a simple mathematical equation that we must keep in mind. I am not sharing this to cause stress rather; to show you that you are in control of your weight loss journey.

How to Develop and Maintain a Healthy Diet Without Dieting

In diet culture, hunger is seen as an enemy. When it comes to intuitive eating, hunger is not an enemy but rather a source of information for you regarding what your body is asking for and what it needs. Instead of seeing hunger as an enemy, I want you to begin listening to your hunger. The philosophy behind this is that if you wait until you are too hungry before you eat, you will be much more likely to overeat because you will feel ravenous and want to eat everything in sight. If, instead, you choose to adhere to your hunger and eat when your body tells you that it needs sustenance, you will be much more likely to eat just the right amount, and you and your body will be satisfied rather than completely stuffed afterward. Instead of feeling shameful and angry that you are feeling hungry, feel happy that your body is telling you what it needs and that you can provide it with nutrients for it to keep working hard for you!

The above concept is how you can lose weight and begin to eat healthier without following a diet or giving in to any diet culture norms proven to be very harmful to people's mental health.

The diet industry may seem like it is in place to help you improve your life and become a better version of yourself, when in fact, it is banking on the fact that you never find success, as this will keep you coming back to spend more money and buy more books. When it comes to being healthy and taking good care of your body, intuitive eating cannot be thought of in the same way as a diet can, it should instead be seen as a philosophy that aims to help you return to the normal way that humans are meant to eat.

The diet industry is focused on making you feel like you are not perfect enough. Taking an approach focused on perfection leaves you feeling down on yourself and like a failure most of the time. Since this method leaves you feeling as though you are always short of perfection (instead of focusing on the positives), the progress you have made will always feel like it is still not enough, no matter how far you have come or how much progress you have made. Since you will never achieve perfection- as this is impossible for anyone, you will never feel satisfaction or celebrate your achievements. You will forever be chasing the "right diet" when, in fact, there is no right diet.

Intuitive eating, as discussed in the previous chapter, can be seen as the anti-diet mentality!

How to Shift Your Mind Toward Weight Loss

Intuitive eating is a good choice for anyone, especially for those who prefer more flexibility when it comes to their eating time and those who do not want to restrict their eating at all. Humans should not be putting themselves through boot camp every time they feel hungry, and this method does not adhere to that type of mindset.

One of the reasons that intuitive eating is such a successful and cherished form of eating is that it allows the body to lead the mind in the right direction when seeking out its needs. For example, did you know that your cravings could be giving you much more information than you give them credit for? Below we will look at what your cravings could mean and why this means that you should let your body guide your eating choices.

By beginning to view your life in this way, you will not fight against your body and mind, but instead, learn to work along with them. This change will help you to achieve a sense of harmony.

Chapter 7: Learning to Love Exercise

Exercise is great for your body, your mind, and your overall health. Adding an exercise regime into your life is as important, if not more, than any other measures you take to maintain your health. For this reason, we will spend an entire chapter learning about how to love exercise and make it a regular part of your life! This chapter will learn about the importance of making peace with your body and how you can begin to do this.

The Benefits of Exercise for Your Mental Health

Exercise has been proven to help with various things in life, such as stress, impotence, and mental health. Exercise will help you in your journey to recovery because of how it affects the different systems of your body. As you know, all of our body systems work together to form the person that we are. If one of them isn't functioning quite as well as it should be, all of the other systems feel the negative effects.

Exercise works on all of your body systems simultaneously. If one of them isn't firing on all cylinders, exercise will help that system feel better because the movement is nothing but healthy for the mind and body.

Exercising will help you take your mind off those nagging cravings and give you a clearer mind overall with which you can look deep inside at those cravings and the emotional issues that are causing them. Exercise will help in all aspects of your life and will help you to continue reaching for recovery.

In addition to this, exercise has positive chemical effects on our minds. When we exercise, our brain releases chemicals that tell us that we enjoy the exercise's effects. This feeling is known as "runner's high," and it is that thrill you feel after you run a long-distance or complete a workout. When you are feeling down and exercise, your mood will lift because of this runner's high. For this reason, it is not so important what kind of physical exercise you do, but rather the fact that you engage in it regularly to help you feel motivated and to keep your mood positive. This runner's high can be compared to those rewarded feelings that the highly sugary foods give us, but with runner's high, the feeling of joy and accomplishment last way longer than the rewarded happy feelings we get from eating food. Industrial food makes our brains feel happy, but our body feels heavy and sluggish. As I mentioned, exercise makes all of our body parts feel great simultaneously, which is why the effects of runner's high are so long-lasting.

How to Begin Using Exercise to Your Benefit

Whether you are a seasoned exerciser or someone who has never exercised before, there is an exercise routine out there for you. Do not be discouraged by your experience level when it comes to exercise, as everyone can benefit from it, and everyone must start somewhere. Do not be discouraged by your experience level when it comes to exercise, as everyone can benefit from it, and everyone must start somewhere. This section will give you several ideas for exercise, no matter the experience level you bring with you, by teaching you about something called *intuitive movement*.

What Is Intuitive Movement?

Intuitive movement is the practice of moving according to the needs and wishes of your body. It can be thought of similarly to intuitive eating, except with the movement of your body instead.

Many people begin following some type of exercise plan to get in shape or to lose weight. This method does not often lead to success, as people often have to try to force themselves to perform exercise that doesn't feel good for their body, which has not been personalized for them, and which they find no enjoyment in. This determination often lasts for a week or two, after which the person becomes fed up and decides that having to push themselves to perform the exercise plan is not worth the potential benefits.

On the other hand, intuitive movement involves a deeper motivation and an enjoyment factor not often present in other kinds of exercise regimes. If you enjoy the movement, you are much more likely to want to perform it, and you will not even need to force your body to do it, as you will genuinely want to take part in it.

There are so many forms of movement available for our bodies, regardless of our skills or experience levels. Below, I will share several types of exercise and their benefits so that you can choose the type of movement that suits you best.

Cardiovascular Exercise Versus Resistance Training

Cardiovascular exercise and resistance training are two different types of exercise that people can benefit from. Cardiovascular exercise is the type of exercise that involves an elevated heart rate due to activities such as running, riding a bicycle, or swimming. This type of exercise is often referred to as "cardio." This type of exercise is usually done for an extended period at a steady state.

Resistance training is a type of exercise that involves using weights to build up your muscles by doing things like squats, push-ups, bicep curls, and so on. This exercise is the type of exercise you would often do if you go to a gym to exercise. Contrary to popular belief, this type of exercise will not make you bulky and muscular, especially if you are a woman. Instead, it will give you more tone and a leaner body.

When we engage in cardiovascular exercise, our heart rate increases; what this does is carry more oxygen to our muscles so that they can keep exercising. It also carries more oxygen to our brain. More oxygen and blood flow to the brain means that your brain will work more efficiently, more sharply, and with more clarity, after you finish exercising. More blood flow to the brain also means that it will be generally healthier. Exercising often and for a continuous period helps keep the brain structures themselves healthy and in working order. Exercise helps with memory, decision making, and learning. Exercise is the most effective antidepressant. Many pills are prescribed to treat and beat depression, but the most effective and most natural way to continually boost your mood and keep it up is through exercise. The effects that exercise has on the brain are far-reaching and numerous.

When we exercise, we become stronger, faster, and more agile. These benefits not only help us to exercise better but it helps us in our everyday lives. Moving through life with more ease than before is a great feeling that can only be achieved through exercise. Our bodies are built to move, and they love it when we do move! Our bodies are built to continually become stronger with the more we do, and this is what inevitably happens as soon as we begin exercising regularly.

You can begin to see aesthetic changes as well. You can see your muscles growing, your body toning, and your fast disappearing. These changes on the inside and outside make us feel great about the body we live in and the progress we are making mentally.

Taking the time to exercise and stick with an exercise regime shows our body that we are willing to do the hard work that exercising takes, and it also shows our mind the same thing.

The Benefits of Other Kinds of Exercise

Numerous other exercises do not fit into one of the two categories as described above. These include exercises such as yoga, Pilates, high-intensity interval training, group training classes, and so on. While these are not considered traditional exercise methods, they are no less valid than resistance training or cardiovascular exercise. Many people who are not too enthused about exercise wish to pursue methods that incorporate more social aspects or slower movements. If this is what you prefer, this is just as valid as going for a run!

There are even more ways to be active such as pursuing activities like gardening, dancing, hiking, kayaking, etc. Any activity that gets your heart rate raised and brings you a sense of joy and accomplishment can be used as an exercise combined with a diet change to bring you weight loss results!

If you normally don't do much exercise or walk around often, begin by taking the stairs sometimes. Begin by deciding to walk some places, like down the street or around the block. Beginning with this type of movement will get your body used to moving again and will get your muscles and joints moving smoothly.

If you occasionally walk, like to a bus stop or the store on your lunch break, you can begin with a little bit more exercise than someone who is sedentary. Since your muscles and joints are likely somewhat used to being in a standing position, you can begin to jog a little bit. You can jog after dinner around the block a few times or jog to the store and walk back every few days. You could also take a yoga class if you wish or do some video-guided yoga at home.

If you have a moderate level of walking in your life and occasionally speed up to a jog, you can begin to move your body around in new and different ways. Try doing sit-ups and push-ups at home before or after your run or run to the park and use the playground equipment to do some chin-ups, some two-foot jumps onto a step, or run up and down the steps a few times. Doing this will keep your heart rate up and teach your body new ways of moving while allowing your upper body muscles to get a bit of attention as well.

If you run frequently and have some bodyweight exercise sessions now and again, try visiting a gym and doing some more weight exercises. You can try squatting, pressing some things overhead, and maybe some bicep curls. Doing this will challenge your muscles in ways that your body weight cannot and take you to a new level of fitness and mood-boosting.

If you are an experienced runner, you are likely quite familiar with the feeling of runner's high. You are likely quite familiar with how exercise can change your mood and take you from feeling hopeless to hopeful. If you want to try some new forms of exercise, try creating a routine in the gym lifting weights. Doing this will take your running to new heights and will give you a new type of exercise experience to break up the running days.

Suppose you are experienced when it comes to exercise, good for you! Continue to challenge yourself in new ways and teach your body new ways of moving. Exercise does nothing but good things, so keep up your routine.

Since exercising helps women regain some of the muscle mass lost due to age, it can be greatly beneficial for women to exercise into their older years. It is important to be aware of how to do this safely, though. It can be safer to stick to low-impact exercises, so exercises that avoid jumping or any sort of quick, jarring movements. Instead, spending some time on an exercise bike (or a real bike) or elliptical machine can be good as they reduce impact and are therefore better for a woman's joints. Things like running involve more impact, so if you have joint pain, it is best to avoid this type of exercise. Further, lifting some small weights or walking with weights in your hands can help you build back some muscle. Building muscle will lead to an increase in your resting rate of metabolism (the number of calories your body burns when it is just sitting, at rest to execute living functions such as breathing or sitting). The increase will greatly improve your overall health in muscle, improve your joint health, and the lowered risk of diseases such as heart disease (which is reduced by doing aerobic exercise). Staying active in your 50's is a great decision, and every capable woman should add exercise into their lives, regardless of the diet they follow.

How Exercise Can Change Your Relationship With Your Body

Exercise meets you where you are, and your brain will gladly take any new form of movement as a mood booster. When you enjoy the exercises that you are taking part in, you are much more likely to choose to engage in them more often and much less likely to find excuses to avoid them. By enjoying what you are doing, it will feel like a reward and not like a punishment. For this reason, be sure to choose a form of exercise (or multiple forms) that you enjoy.

Exercising while on this process to recovery will help you feel strong both physically and mentally when your journey may be getting tough. Exercising will show you what your body can do, and how strong it is, making you feel stronger mentally.

The Importance of Sleep

You may have heard before that sleep is essential to a person's success in every aspect of their life, but you may not know why this is. A person's sleep cycle has been proven to have strong effects on their mood and their willpower. When a person does not get enough sleep, their symptoms of depression, or their negative mood, in general, have been shown to worsen.

Sleep deprivation causes other negative symptoms like sadness, fatigue, moodiness, and irritability. When you are trying to pursue a lifestyle change, including incorporating more exercise and changing your diet, you need to maintain a positive mood to remain motivated and track to accomplish your goals.

Since the theory behind willpower is that it requires energy from the brain to be maintained, and the brain restores its energy from a restful sleep, it's safe to assume that sleep is directly connected to the level of willpower that a person can exercise. When a person doesn't get enough sleep, their brain spends most of its energy focused on keeping the body's basic functions up and running (such as walking, breathing, and moving. These energy demands do not leave much energy for a person to spend on exerting their willpower, practicing self-discipline, or simply remembering their goals.

Getting a proper and healthy amount of sleep is vital for accomplishing anything, especially if those things are challenging. When a person doesn't get enough sleep, it affects their ability to focus, judgment, mood, overall health, and diet.

When people suffer chronic sleep deprivation such as insomnia, things go from bad to worse. Many research studies have found evidence that people who don't get the proper amount of sleep regularly have a greater risk of catching specific diseases. Lack of sleep also has a significant and negative impact on a person's immune system. This impact can cause a person to frequently catch colds or flu cases that cause them not to go to school, work, or get anything effective done.

Not many people can function well with less than seven hours of sleep per night. A healthy adult should be aiming for 7 – 9 hours of sleep every night. For an adult, it is important to get at least six hours of sleep every night. A healthy amount of sleep should range between eight to ten hours every night, but the minimum requirement is 6 hours. To ensure you are getting this much sleep, avoid eating or drinking anything that contains caffeine for at least 5 hours before bedtime so that it doesn't affect your natural sleep cycle. Make a note to also stay away from ingesting too many toxins during the day such as cigarettes, alcohol, drugs, or prescription medicine if it can be avoided, as these can lead to a reduction in sleep quality.

The benefits of getting enough sleep are extraordinary. Aside from the fact that it can help you stay focused and be more disciplined, it also helps with the following;

- curbing inflammation and pain
- lowering stress
- improving your memory
- jumpstarting your creativity

- sharpening your attention
- improving your grades
- limiting your chances of accidents
- helping you avoid negative feelings that can lead to depression or anxiety.

Chapter 8: Using Affirmations

This chapter will learn about a great strategy that will prove useful to you in helping you reach your weight loss goals. This tool can help you because of the positive mental state that it can put you in, and because of the increase in self-esteem it can bring you. This tool is something called an *Affirmation*.

What Are Affirmations?

Affirmations are, by definition, spoken or written phrases, which state something to be true. More specifically, affirmations are the valuable and uplifting assurances that we tell ourselves. They are words or phrases that we use to state something about ourselves or our lives to be true.

Declarations are similar to affirmations in that they are the act of declaring something. The difference between affirmations and declarations is that declarations can be an opinion or a belief rather than a fact. The word declaration can be used as a noun or as a verb, as in *to make a declaration*, which is when you share your declaration with others in the form of writing or speaking.

We will look at some examples of affirmations and declarations below, and I will teach you how to make some for yourself to use in your own life. Please note that from here forward, we can use the terms affirmation and declaration interchangeably.

How Affirmations Will Benefit You

The technique of implementing change that lasts is to change the way someone perceives themselves. So how does affirmation play a role here? Affirmations are very effective when used out loud so that you can hear the positive reminders being said in your voice. Humans naturally believe the things that they tell themselves. For example, if someone dislikes some aspect of their physical appearance, they will believe that they are unattractive. The next time you are in front of a mirror, practice using affirmations by saying something you like about yourself. By repeating this every time, you are in front of a mirror will eventually lead you to believe these positive things, and you will begin to focus on the positive rather than what you don't like about yourself.

How to Use Affirmations

If someone is trying to improve their self-esteem or their negative mind state, the affirmations they use should be focused solely on positive things.

Suppose a person wishes to use affirmations to achieve specific goals. In that case, it is beneficial for them to use affirmations that remind them of their positive personal values and their potential.

Try repeating your affirmations aloud to yourself, or even writing them down (or better yet, a combination of both) frequently. Doing this will help you build a positive self-narrative that will lead to an increase in your level of self-esteem over time and, thus, a greater likelihood of achieving your goals.

We will look at the steps you will need to take to create your own affirmations below, and once you have created them for yourself, you will be ready to begin using them right away. Once you have completed your positive affirmations, schedule a block of time every day or a couple of times per week to take a look back at them and update them. The more you read them and drill them into your memory, the more positive thoughts will naturally come to you. You can also document any changes you feel in yourself as you do this exercise.

How to Come up With Affirmations of Your Own

1. **Structure your affirmation** To begin, you want to structure your affirmation
so that it begins with something called an *"I statement."* This point means that you want to start your sentence with *"I am..."*

2. **Focus on creating affirmations that have a positive outcome**.
Try to refrain from using avoidant words such as "not" in your statements. Make them as positive as you can, as your brain feels positive when it hears positive words like "can!"

3. **Keep your affirmations as concise as you can.**

Ensure they are concise, so they guide you to the point and serve as quick reminders of positivity.

4. **Design your affirmations to be as specific as possible**.

This point is especially important if it guides you to your goal, as you want to ensure that you are keeping yourself focused on the goal so that you are continuously reminding yourself of it.

5. **Try to write your affirmations in the present tense**.

Focus on using a word that ends with "ing" this will help you ensure that you are using the word's present tense.

6. **Use descriptive words**

Using descriptive words will give your affirmation more impact and will make it more detailed.

7. **Make your affirmations personal to you and your situation**.

Ensure that your affirmations relate to your specific goals or whatever you are dealing with at the moment; this will increase their impact when you use them and help you remember why you are using them.

Chapter 9: Hypnosis Techniques for Weight Loss

In this chapter, we will discuss the topic of hypnosis and how it can benefit you in this weight loss journey that you are embarking on.

What Is Hypnosis?

Hypnosis is the practice of reaching an altered state of consciousness where a person is said to lose control of their actions and is very susceptible to the power of suggestion or to being given direction. This technique is done to achieve new behaviors or thoughts that were previously difficult to grasp or understand. This method is also done to break tough habits or addictions, such as an addiction to smoking cigarettes.

This practice works because this altered state of consciousness allows a person to become more open-minded and receptive to suggestions. Without hypnosis, a person may be resistant to accepting new thoughts or concepts, and they may be closed off to new ideas or trying new behaviors. If these are introduced in a hypnosis state, the person will be much more open to them, and when they return to a normal state of consciousness, they will be left with these imprinted ideas, beliefs, or behaviors. This method works because it taps into the subconscious mind, where the conscious mind cannot step in and inhibit the absorption of concepts or ideas that it decides it does not want. By programming these new ideas and thoughts into the subconscious mind, your body can act according to thoughts you are unaware of, and this is how new beliefs or behaviors can come about before you can stop them.

The altered state of consciousness achieved by undergoing hypnosis is similar to the state that is achieved in the moments before a person falls asleep. In these moments, a person is said to be the most creative, relaxed, and open-minded.

The Benefits Of Hypnosis

Hypnosis has proven beneficial for removing negative beliefs or thought patterns, including limiting beliefs and replacing them with new positive or beneficial beliefs. This practice is especially effective for those stubborn and deep-seated beliefs and habits that you have been trying to kick but have been unable to. Since you now understand that deep emotional struggles often cause weight gain and obesity, you can see how hypnosis can help a person overcome those struggles and lose weight for good.

In addition to the above benefits, hypnosis has been shown to reduce pain, reduce anxiety, and bring about a sense of calm to a person. It can also improve your sleep quality and improve Irritable Bowel Syndrome (IBS) symptoms, which affects a large portion of the population.

For our specific purposes, hypnosis is beneficial for several reasons. It allows a person to become receptive to the power of suggestion; it can help a person cast off their negative self-image and see themselves positively.

Further, it can help break the cycle of emotional eating by dealing with the root causes of this type of eating and can teach a person to turn to different methods of dealing with their feelings and emotions other than turning to food. This conscious choice can break the cycle of emotional eating; as I said in the previous chapter, the most effective way to deal with this is to examine the root causes and address those first. As this is very difficult to do for many people, especially if the root causes are painful to revisit, hypnosis can effectively access those deep feelings and fears to confront and deal with them. Hypnosis does this by removing the mental blocks that the conscious mind puts up to protect us from our negative feelings and fears.

There are three ways that you can change your emotional state whenever you wish to. These ways include changing yourself on a physical level, on a mental level, and finally, using verbal techniques. We will look at each of these three ways in more detail below, including how hypnosis can benefit you in each of these three ways.

1. Physical

Hypnosis works at the physical level by helping you relax your body using deep breathing and a lowered cognition level.

2. Mental

Hypnosis works to change your emotional state as it allows you to change your thought patterns, which changes your emotional state

   3. Verbal

To change your emotional state using verbal techniques, you must employ methods such as the following
- Changing the words you use from negative to positive ones
- Listening to guided meditations (hypnosis) as a way to learn to employ new vocabulary

The Different Levels Of Consciousness

Hypnosis allows a person to reach different levels of consciousness that they otherwise may not be able to. You may be wondering what different levels of consciousness are possible with the human mind.

The Conscious Mind

The conscious mind includes everything that you are aware of. This state includes your thoughts, your short-term memories, and anything that is currently occupying your mind.

The Subconscious Mind

On the other hand, the subconscious mind is the part of your consciousness without your knowledge. This level includes things like memories, which are in your mind which you are not currently aware of, but which can be brought into your conscious mind any time you wish to access them.

The 5 Levels Of Consciousness

When it comes to hypnosis, there are considered to be five levels of consciousness. These different states of consciousness represent different levels of use of the conscious and the subconscious mind.

1. Gamma

The Gamma level of consciousness is that which is entered when brain activity is very high. This state includes times of fear, panic, and anxiety when thoughts in the conscious mind are running quickly from one to the next.

2. Beta

The Beta level of consciousness is the regular state of consciousness that you are in most of the time throughout your life. This stage includes a regular level of awareness of what you are doing and thinking and a regular brain activity level.

3. Alpha

Alpha level of consciousness can be said to be a *Daydream*-like state of mind. This level can be the early stages of hypnosis or when you are meditating. This level begins to include the subconscious mind.

4. Theta

This level is when the subconscious mind begins to take over. There is little conscious thought involved at this level, and you are in touch with the subconscious. This level is usually found during sleep and deeper states of meditation and hypnosis.

    5. Delta

The fifth and final level of consciousness is the Delta level. This level is the deepest, and it does not involve any conscious mind, and it involves a state of deep sleep or a deep trance. This state can be achieved during the deepest sleep levels or by people skilled and experienced with meditation and hypnosis.

How Can Hypnosis Help With Weight Loss?

Hypnosis effectively changes a person's body because it opens the mind to accepting and practicing new behaviors. By changing behaviors, a person can change their body. These behaviors include eating habits and exercise habits. Further, hypnosis can lead to release from negative thought patterns and negative body image. In turn, this practice can also lead to a reduction in the likelihood of emotional eating, as the mind and body will not be seeking comfort and feelings of reward like they were when the person's mind was wrought with negativity.

One of the first beliefs that we want to change through hypnosis is the negative beliefs that you have about your weight.

We want to address and change through hypnosis because of the negative beliefs you hold about weight loss and dieting and the negative beliefs you have about exercise.

We want to replace these negative beliefs with new positive and empowering ones so that you can begin to change your life as a whole.

Hypnosis For Cravings

Below we will look at how you can begin to change the negative thought processes that occur in your mind and how you can begin to reshape them to develop a new perspective of weight loss and diet using hypnosis.

By taking stock of your unhelpful thinking styles and your core wounds, you will begin to notice them as they come up in your mind throughout the day. By being able to do this, you can begin to turn them around by consciously combatting them and reminding yourself of your positive thinking styles. This practice will help you remain on track to achieving your goals and making this new lifestyle a habit. By doing this during the day, you are training your mind to reach for positive thoughts instead of negative ones over time. Eventually, those positive thoughts will happen more often than the unhelpful ones. This type is a form of self-hypnosis, as you are changing your beliefs and thoughts, which is one of the main goals of hypnosis.

Suppose you can get yourself into a daydream-like state several times during the day and, from there, shift your thinking toward positivity and goal-oriented thoughts. In that case, you can begin to allow your subconscious to feed you those positive thoughts throughout the day, which will help with your motivation and your daily pursuit of your weight loss and diet goals. By catching and changing your thoughts before they spiral out of control, you will be in control of your emotions and behavior as well.

By intervening in your natural thought progression when it comes to weight loss, you can change your thoughts regarding weight-loss into more positive and goal-oriented thoughts. For example, instead of thinking, "I will fail at weight loss because I always have in the past," You can instead jump in and change this automatic negative thought to something more positive. For example, "This time, I will succeed since I have set myself up for success by goal setting and reading this book." During hypnosis, you can change your negative fail-focused thoughts to more positive ones, which will lead these positive thoughts to come to the surface more readily in your daily life after that. Doing this will, in turn, inform your behavior and lead you to success.

Doing this can help you deal with nagging cravings because you can consciously choose to avoid them and instead make a healthier choice for yourself.

Self-Hypnosis

Self-Hypnosis, in contrast to other types of hypnotherapy, is done alone rather than with a therapist or a "hypnotizer" present. Self-hypnosis is done by getting yourself into a state of deep relaxation, to the point of allowing the subconscious mind to come to the surface and encouraging the conscious mind to take a back seat. When you get into a self-hypnosis state, you can then begin to introduce the suggestion portion of hypnosis- either in the form of suggesting new thoughts and behaviors to yourself or by listening to an audio guide for this exact purpose. These audioguides can be found online in a variety of places, one of which is YouTube. With self-hypnosis, you can use any form of hypnosis that you wish (any of those described above), according to the motivations for using hypnosis in the first place.

If you are just getting started with self-hypnosis, the best way to initiate this is by practicing mindfulness. We discussed mindfulness briefly in this book thus far, but here I will show you an example of how you can get into a state of mindfulness to begin self-hypnosis if you are not experienced with it.

Mindfulness and meditation go hand in hand. Meditation increases mindfulness while mindfulness improves and deepens meditation. Meditation is a practice, while mindfulness is a state of being.

To get into a state of mindfulness involves getting quiet and observing, without judgment, everything that occurs within your body. You must let your thoughts drift by, noticing but not judging them. Notice all of your body's physical feelings; is there any tension that you notice? Notice how breathing feels on a physical level. Feel any sensations that you are experiencing. Notice also your emotions and feelings. By doing this repeatedly, you will be able to eventually focus on your body with less and less distracting thoughts. When your thoughts start to distract you, bring your attention back to your body, and breathing. Being able to reach a state like this allows you to reconnect with your body from the inside. Approaching your body with a non-judgment mindset will also make it easier for you to change your beliefs about your body or introduce new thoughts and behaviors. Instead of letting your mind spiral with anxious *what-if* thoughts, you will not let them escalate. They will not escalate to the level they normally would because instead of judging yourself and your body and worrying about what is wrong with you, you will approach it as is and without trying to force anything.

By focusing on the body and letting your thoughts enter your consciousness one by one, you can untangle them, resulting in a reduction in stress level. The state of meditation also brings about a state of relaxation and calm. Often, we are running around with a mind full of running thoughts, one after the other. When we take time to sit in silence, breathe, and sort through everything we are thinking and feeling through a non-judgmental lens, it leads to a state of inner peace. This inner peace state makes it much easier for your body to let in and embrace the good feelings and allows your mind to be more open and receptive to them.

By trying this exercise several times, it will begin to come easier over time, and you will then be able to get into a state of self-hypnosis much quicker. Once you have reached this level, you can then practice any sort of hypnosis in the form of self-hypnotism.

Other Techniques

When it comes to hypnosis, there are a variety of different types that you can engage in. In this section, I will outline them to get a better idea of how they can be employed in your life to help you in your journey of self-discovery and weight loss.

- Cognitive Hypnotherapy

The first type of hypnotherapy that we will discuss is called *cognitive hypnotherapy*. The term *hypnotherapy* relates to hypnosis therapy, and these two terms (hypnotherapy and hypnosis) can be used interchangeably.

Cognitive hypnotherapy is a type of hypnosis that is focused on a person's beliefs. It aims to change these beliefs to free a person from their limiting beliefs. It encourages people to look at their lives and beliefs from a new perspective and re-evaluate them. This type of hypnosis is similar in many ways to traditional Cognitive Behavioral Therapy (CBT), a type of talk therapy used to treat people with a variety of mental health disorders that includes depression, anxiety, as well as PTSD (Post-Traumatic Stress Disorder). CBT's fundamentals are based on three components; cognition (thought), emotion, and behavior. All three components interact with each other in the human mind, which leads to the theory that our thoughts determine our feelings and emotions, which then determines our behavior. Again, this is further evidence of the mind-body connection at work. Cognitive Behavioral Therapy works by emphasizing the relationship between your thoughts, feelings, and behaviors. When you begin to change any of these three components, you begin to initiate change in the other two components. CBT aims to increase your life's overall quality by helping you examine it from a new perspective. In this way, cognitive hypnotherapy can be beneficial for our purposes here, as it aims to change behaviors through changing thoughts or addressing emotions.

- Behavioral Hypnotherapy

This type of hypnotherapy is one of the classic forms, as it is one of the first practiced hypnotherapies. This type of hypnotherapy is a great place to begin if a person has no hypnotherapy experience. It is less intrusive and mentally demanding than some other forms of hypnotherapy. As you can guess, this type is done to change people's behaviors by shifting the current behaviors to more positive ones. The therapist will get the patient into a state of hypnosis. Then they will begin to suggest and talk through alternative behaviors to introduce them into the person's subconscious mind, therefore solidifying them for the person.

- Regression Hypnotherapy

Regression hypnotherapy is one of the more demanding and intrusive types of hypnotherapy. It involves looking back into a person's memories in their subconscious mind to tackle the root causes of whatever problems or struggles the person is having. This kind of therapy relates to what we discussed in the first chapter of this book, where we looked at possible underlying causes of a negative internal environment.

By taking part in regression hypnotherapy, a person can revisit their past or childhood to determine what types of trauma or events led them to develop the problems they are looking to overcome.

This type of hypnotherapy is not done until a person is comfortable with the practice of hypnosis, and it comes with some risks, as it could lead a person to be re-traumatized. This practice should only be done with a therapist whom you trust and only after experiencing other hypnosis forms.

Visualization As A Form Of Self-Hypnosis

In this section, we will look at visualization and how this can come together with hypnosis to influence the mind, and therefore the body (thanks to the mind-body connection) to make lasting changes for the better.

What Is Visualization?

Most people have tried to visualize their goals at least a couple of times in their lives. They probably spend a lot of time visualizing a desired future event. For the general public, visualization is a process where they picture their future within their mind. However, visualization can be used for much more than just that. It is a type of inner transformation that leads to seeing actual results in reality. Visualization is also a form of creative thinking where people can shape their lives using a specific purpose within their minds. The best part about the image is that a person may have envisioned that it doesn't have to rely upon the outer world's external events. It can depend entirely on a person's imagination.

The Benefits Of Visualization

Here is something that not many people know: Visualizing an action or a skill before actually performing it is nearly as effective as physically doing it. Scientific studies found evidence of people's thoughts creating the exact same patterns of activity in their mind as it does with the physical movements of the action. When somebody is mentally rehearsing or practicing something in their mind using the visualization process, it impacts the many cognitive processes within a person's brain, including planning, motor control, memory, and attention perception. In layman's terms, the way a person's brain is stimulated when they visualize an action is the same as when they are performing it physically. Therefore, scientists can safely assume that the act of visualization provides just as much value as physically performing a task.

Many athletes in certain sports use the act of visualization to help themselves train before a competition. For example, in Olympic cycling, the cyclist will prepare for a competition by closing their eyes and visualizing the racetrack in their mind. They move their bodies while visualizing how they will travel through the racetrack to train their muscle memory and reflexes even further. This way, when they do begin to compete on the racetrack, they have already visualized themselves cycling through it using the strategies that they have been taught and visualized in their minds. This technique is a technique and training skill that many professional coaches teach their athletes to do.

When a person is visualizing, their conscious mind is aware that what they're visualizing is not real but is just a result of imagination. Consequently, a person's subconscious cannot differentiate the difference between what a person is thinking and what they are doing. In other words, a person's inner mind isn't able to distinguish the difference between real life, a photo, memories, or an imagined future. Rather, the mind is under the impression that everything a person sees is real. This fact is proven by numerous brain scans that scientists have conducted over the years. They discovered that there are no brain activity differences when someone observes something in the real world compared to when a person is visualizing.

All of this evidence is extremely important because it points to the theory that visualization can help people learn new skills and reprogram and rewire their brains without performing physical actions. For example, suppose somebody is looking to increase their self-esteem. In that case, they can use visualization by imagining themselves doing those actions before actually doing it in the real world.

How To Use Visualization

Below, I will outline several different examples of visualization practice that you can try in various scenarios. These visualization exercises can help you create an action plan to help you achieve your goals or begin putting a plan into action before taking physical action to achieve goals you have set out for yourself already.

Visualization for Creating a Plan of Action

It is normal to become stressed out or feel overwhelmed when trying to achieve new goals. For this reason, creating a plan of action using visualization can help you relax and motivate you to take action. This technique is most effective if you use it before you go to bed to start planning the next day. You can also use this technique anytime during the day, when you have 10 minutes of free time.

Below are three simple steps on how to do this:

1. Calm yourself down and make sure you are feeling relaxed. Sit down as it will help you get some rest from whatever you were doing before.
2. Close your eyes and start to visualize which things specifically that you want to accomplish for tomorrow. Now, visualize those actions that you'd like to do in as much detail as you can and then ask yourself these questions below:

    a) How would I like to feel?
    b) How may I act around others?
    c) Which specific actions do I want to take?
    d) What do I want?
    e) Which challenges may I face?
    f) How can I deal with these challenges?
    g) What results do I want to come from this?

3. The reality here is that people cannot predict all the things that might happen to them. When events happen unexpectedly, they can often ruin any plans that have been put in place. However, good planning isn't about planning around all possible obstacles, but it is more about adapting to the obstacles that life gives you. When you keep this in mind, you must affirm with yourself at the end of

your session with "this or something better will come my way." By giving yourself affirmation, you are keeping your mind open to endless possibilities. This practice will result in more ready and okay with making adjustments when unexpected things happen to you.

This process is not a foolproof plan. However, this visualization will help you envision possible situations that might happen. These scenarios will help you choose more ideal options for yourself as you continue to work towards your goals.

Visualization for Achieving Goals That You Have Set Out for Yourself

This visualization technique is the most important one when it comes to strengthening self-discipline. Using the visualization technique for setting goals brings a lot of value, but this technique does come with one major drawback. The most popular form of visualization is goal setting. Most people have used visualization pertaining to their goals at one time or another. However, this technique may not have worked for them due to one critical flaw. This flaw is that when people visualize their goals, they only focus on visualizing their end goal and nothing in between. They see within their mind's a big and flashy awesome goal that's going to be rainbows and butterflies. Yes, they are experiencing this using all of their senses, but they simply open their eyes after the visualization, feeling very inspired. However, this type of motivation is extremely short-lived because the next time this person faces an obstacle, it immediately deflates their motivation.

When this happens, people feel the imagine the same goal all over again to create extra motivation. Though, because nothing happens after visualizing again, their motivation does not grow either. In fact, every time a person hits an obstacle and tries the process of visualization again, their motivation becomes weaker every time, and they start to lose more and more energy.

The mistake that these people are making is that they are not properly visualizing their goals. They only see the destination, but they don't understand that achieving a goal takes much more than just that. Achieving a goal is part of a journey that is full of emotional highs and lows, wins and losses, and journey of ups and downs. Due to this, these are the things that a person would also need to include in their visualization.

When a person visualizes their end goal, it is very effective in creating that desire and hunger. However, the proper way to use visualization is to spend 10 percent of your time visualizing the end goal and spending the rest of the visualization time thinking about HOW you will achieve your goals and overcome challenges. In some ways, it's similar to the form of visualization planning that we just discussed.

A person's end goal helps keep inspiration running in the long term, but it is the journey that helps a person stay motivated in the short term. To maximize the time spent on achieving small goals to get to your end goal, you must visualize those as well.

Below are five steps that you can follow to achieve this visualization:
1. Get yourself to a quiet place and sit down and close your eyes. Start to visualize the final stage of your goals. Imagine that you are experiencing and living the new reality that achieving your goal will bring you, using each of your five senses.
2. Slowly take steps backward from the end goal by visualizing the steps that you would take to achieve your end goal. Imagine the problems you might need to overcome; imagine yourself overcoming them. Picture yourself finding solutions to those problems. Continue visualizing until you reach the moment you are currently living.
3. Next, fast-forward from this moment and imagine which actions helped you overcome your problems.
4. After you finish this visualization, spend a few moments sending your future self some positive vibes and wish them luck on their journey.
5. When you exit the visualization, emotionally detach from the outcome of your goal. One factor that could potentially inhibit you is to having an emotional tie to a particular outcome. Alternatively, try to remain open-

minded, flexible and receptive to whatever is to come on your journey.

You can use visualization using those steps on a daily or weekly basis. Weekly sessions can be as long as 30 minutes, and you can keep your daily sessions shorter, so they are between 5 - 10 minutes. However, be sure that you are using your daily sessions to visualize the next steps on your journey to achieving the goals over the upcoming week. Doing this helps a person to continue making progress towards reaching their goal. After that, you can use your weekly visualizations using the five steps above.

Chapter 10: Motivation

In this chapter, we will look at the all-important and very difficult concept of motivation. First, I will define the term motivation for you, and then we will begin looking at how to find and maintain motivation to keep pursuing your new lifestyle.

What Is Motivation?

Motivation is different for every person. Motivation is different in every area of life, but it is possible to reduce motivation to one single definition.

Motivation is something within a person that drives them towards a wish to change something about their life. These desired changes can be internal (mental, emotional, etc.) or external (in a person's environment). Motivation comes down to wanting to achieve, attain, or accomplish something that you do not have. Motivation combines the desire to change with the desired direction to make a person take action and steps toward the outcomes they want.

Motivation is what helps people accomplish things that they set out to do. For this reason, when trying to accomplish something difficult and challenging, you will search for motivation because it will help you reach your goals.

Now that you understand motivation on a deeper level, we will look at finding and maintaining motivation.

How To Find Motivation

To better understand motivation and how it comes about, we will look at the science behind it.

Some motivation is triggered by needs that you do not even think about, like the need to sustain your life by eating, sleeping, and having connections. Simultaneously, some motivation is triggered by the needs of a psychological nature, such as the need to have a meaningful human connection. To better understand this, we will look at the research of one particular psychologist. Abraham Maslow was a psychologist who specialized in human needs and who came up with a list of human needs that every person seeks to have met. These needs that he researched were broken up into different categories, and within each of these categories are several needs. We will look at these needs below to gain a better understanding of what these categories entail.

Physiological Needs
This category houses the most basic set of needs and includes human needs for survival such as;
- Water
- Air
- Shelter
- Food
- Clothing
- Sleep
- Sex

Safety

This set of needs is the next most basic, but they become a little more abstract in this set than the previous group's physical needs. These needs include;
- Good health
- Employment
- Personal security
- Property
- Resources

Love & Belonging
This set of needs is where it becomes less about what humans need to survive with their basic requirements taken care of and more about those emotional needs. This set of needs includes;
- Family
- Friendship
- Intimacy
- A sense of human connection

Self-Esteem
In this section, this is that set of needs that not everyone can have met in their life, but if you are lucky enough to have these met, you are more privileged than most people on earth. These needs are not extras, as they are still considered human needs, but unfortunately, they are not available to everyone. These needs are;
- Status
- Respect
- Recognition
- Self-esteem
- Freedom
- Strength

Self-Actualization
This section only involves one need, and this single need gives the section its namesake;
- Self-actualization, or the desire to reach one's full potential in every sense of the word.

When it comes to the needs involved in Maslow's findings, you will easily find the motivation to perform tasks that bring you closer to having these needs met. That is because these needs are programmed into every person when they are born, and we spend our lives seeking to fulfill them.

On the other hand, when you are looking to fulfill goals such as; making lots of money, getting a six-pack, or practicing yoga every day for a year, it will be much more difficult to find the motivation to do so. One way around this is to connect your goals to one of the needs in the above lists. For example, say you want to make lots of money. In this case, it may be hard to motivate yourself to pick up an extra job or to stay late at work every night. To combat this, try to connect this want to a human need. In this case, you could say that wanting to make lots of money is connected to a need under the *safety* section, say, property or resources. Alternatively, it could be connected to a need under the *self-esteem* section, say, recognition, or status. It could be connected to any of these needs, or any combination of these needs, depending on the person.

Now, when it comes to the goals that we are discussing in this book, like; losing "x" number of pounds, working out for 30 minutes per day, or cutting out 80% of the sugar from your diet, think about what needs those goals could be connected to. This answer will be personal for you, so take some time to think about this. Doing this on your own will help you find your motivation, as nobody else can find it for you!

How To Maintain Motivation

By examining your motivations, you will be likely to stay on track. By understanding your personal motivating needs for something, you wish to achieve or accomplish, you will likely remember why you began. You will be likely to keep pushing through when things become difficult during the process.

Self-Judgement And How To Overcome It

Self-judgement is something that everybody deals with to some degree. In this section, we will look at how you can take back the reins when it comes to your thoughts and feelings about yourself and how you can begin to re-shift them.

- Be aware

Awareness is the first step that needs to be taken to recognize your inner-critic and reshape it into something less critical and more supportive. Try to pay attention the next time you are feeling distracted, numb, or anxious. Try to identify whose voice is the voice of your inner critic. Try to find the situation where your inner critic awakens. It allows you to dig deep and identify the most vulnerable feelings during situations where your inner critic is awake. These feelings or these situations are likely what your inner critic is trying to protect you from feeling. However, by protecting you, they are holding you back from meeting your full potential. When people have developed unhelpful thinking processes, it is hard to make decisions to benefit their future self because their thoughts create negative emotions that drive away motivation. Some people argue that by simply increasing your willpower, thus overcoming the need for instant gratification, you will fix your situation. This belief, however, is not an effective solution for long-lasting change. In this section, we will look at a variety of ways that you can begin to combat those limiting beliefs and the negative self-talk that goes on in your mind.

- Remind Yourself To Be Positive

As we learned, bad habits are built through many years, and no amount of willpower can handle overcoming that many bad habits in a person's life. Rewiring your brain to minimize the amount of negativity you feel in the first place is a much more efficient method to approach this problem.

- Catch Yourself Thinking According To Your Limiting Beliefs

Often, if the person had just paid attention to their thought process, they would be able to catch themselves before their mind automatically spiraled to a place of complete de-motivation. By catching yourself before you get there, you can prevent yourself from falling into your negative thought patterns, limiting you and holding you back.

- Show Yourself Evidence Against Your Limiting Belief

Showing yourself evidence that supports or doesn't support the thoughts that are on your mind will help you to change your limiting beliefs. Showing yourself evidence can cancel out those negative thinking styles and give yourself the confidence and motivation to overcome any situation.

If a person is stuck in the mindset that they will fail, saying something like, "Oh, I'm going to fail and embarrass myself anyway, so why prepare?" The majority of the time, people of this mindset will choose not to prepare, thus leading to a feeling of failure when they inevitably do not come prepared for success. This mentality further solidifies their limiting belief.

When your inner critic begins to tell you that you can't do a certain thing, or you're not good enough, or you're not worthy enough, simply find evidence within your past life experiences that challenge or discount this belief. Prove your inner critic wrong and show them why holding you back is only going to do more harm than if you failed whatever task you were planning to do. The more you tell your inner critic this, the more they will learn to listen to you and help you in another way that is not just preventing you from doing things.

- Ask For Support From Your Inner Critic

Suppose your inner-critic is telling you that you will embarrass yourself and everyone will laugh at you. In that case, you can first prove it wrong by using evidence-based arguments, negotiate with it to let you try it out, and then ask for its support by saying, "This is a difficult challenge for me, and I want to overcome it. I need you to be by my side, regardless of the outcome." Remember, your inner critic is just another version of yourself. Be kind to it even if it's not kind to you. Showing kindness to yourself is very important in our case.

- Negotiate With Your Limiting Beliefs To Change Them

When you can notice these voices and statements that are going on in your brain according to your limiting beliefs, you can then simply acknowledge them and begin to negotiate with your inner critic. Let them know that you thank them for looking out for you, but you are confident in your ability to make decisions for yourself. You can let them know that even though you may fail and feel embarrassed, it is still better than a lifetime of holding back. Since your inner critic is a part of you, after all, it can listen to reason as long as you allow yourself to be reasoned with.

- Surround Yourself With Positive People

Surrounding yourself with people that can encourage you and foster positivity will also change your inner-critic's opinion. Often, hearing positive compliments from other people hold a heavier weight in the eyes of your inner-critic compared to you telling your inner-critic the same thing. Try spending time with people who support your goals and the changes you are looking to make in your life. It will make your journey a little bit easier.

Limiting beliefs and negative self-talk and negative body-image can lead a person to feel terrible about themselves, often to the point of feeling like they hate themselves. As I mentioned earlier, to make lasting changes, we will work on loving ourselves instead of hating ourselves. By positively seeing your body, because of all of the things it allows you to do, you will begin to make choices with your body's health in mind. Doing this will lead to lasting, positive changes for your physical and mental health.

- Be gentle with yourself.

It is important to be gentle with ourselves because we are usually our own toughest examiner. We look at ourselves very critically, and we often think that nothing we do is good enough. We must be gentle with ourselves to not discourage ourselves, put ourselves down, or make ourselves feel bad about what we are working hard to accomplish. We must remind ourselves that everything in life is a process and does not happen instantly, and we mustn't tell ourselves to "hurry up and succeed," as we often do.

When you fall off track, you must not beat yourself up for this. It is important to be gentle with yourself. Beating yourself up will only cause you to turn into a spiral of negativity and continue to talk down to yourself. Doing this will make you lose motivation and will make you feel like you are a failure. Having this state of mind will make it difficult not to turn to food for comfort. We must avoid this entire process by avoiding beating ourselves up in the first place. If we don't beat ourselves up and instead encourage ourselves, we will not even make ourselves feel the need to find safety. Instead of thinking of how we can't do it, and it is too hard and then needing to turn to food for comfort and a feeling of safety, we will instead talk to ourselves positively and encourage ourselves from within. Instead of making ourselves feel bad, we will instead feel motivated, and we will be even more ready to continue on our journey.

Even if you don't fall off the plan, it is still important to talk to yourself nicely and encourage. We must recognize that changing our behaviors that we have likely been doing for some time is no small feat. We must encourage ourselves just like we would encourage someone else. Think of it like you are talking to a good friend or family member on this journey instead of you. What would you say to them? How would you say it? You would likely be quite gentle and loving in your words. You would likely tell them that they were doing a great job and keeping it up. This example is exactly how you want to speak to yourself from within and the exact types of words and phrases you want to use. If we spoke to our friends the way we speak to ourselves most of the time, they would be quite hurt. Thus, we must remember this when trying to motivate ourselves, and we must be gentle.

Another way to be gentle with yourself is to avoid being too restrictive in the beginning. You must understand that it will be a challenge, and easing into this new lifestyle will be best. Beginning by making small changes and then adding more and more changes as you go will be a good way for your mind and body to get used to the changes. If you dump many changes on yourself too quickly, this will be quite a challenge for your mind and body.

How to Make Your New Lifestyle a Habit

Now that you have learned a wealth of information about intuitive eating, we will look at some strategies that you can use to make these new, healthy choices a habit. Making this a habit will take time, but you will surely find success by employing these strategies.

This section will look at a real-life example of dealing with challenges to demonstrate healthy thinking patterns when it comes to intuitive eating.

Let's say you are trying to focus on healthy eating, and you have had trouble doing so. Maybe you ate a cupcake, or maybe you had a soda at breakfast. From the perspective of the traditional diet mentality, this would become a problem for the diet, which would become a problem in your mind. You would likely be beating yourself up and feeling terrible about the choice you have made.

Let's look at this example in more detail. It is very important to avoid beating yourself up or self-judging for falling off the wagon. Negative self-talk may happen sometimes. What we need to do to combat this is to not focus on the fact that it has happened but on how we are going to deal with and react to it. There are a variety of reactions that a person may have to this type of situation. We will examine the possible reactions and their pros and cons below:

- You may feel as though your progress is ruined and that you might as well begin another time again. This strategy could lead you to go back to your old ways and keep you from trying again for quite some time. This effect could happen many times, over and over again, and each time you slip up, you decide that you might as well give up this time and try again, but each time it ends the same.

- You may fall off your plan and tell yourself that this day is a write-off and that you will begin the next day again. The problem with this method is that continuing the rest of the day as you would have before you decided to make a change will make it so that the next day is like beginning all over again, and it will be very hard to begin again. You may be able to begin the next day again, and it could be fine, but you must be able to motivate yourself if you are going to do this. Knowing that you have fallen off in the past makes it so that you may feel down on yourself and feel as though you can't do it, so beginning again the next day is very important.

- The third option, similar to the previous case, you may fall off, but instead of deciding that the day is a write-off, you tell yourself that the entire week is a write-off, and you then decide that you will pick it up again the next week. This method will be even harder than starting the next day again, as multiple days of eating whatever you like will make it very hard to go back to making the healthy choices again afterward.

- After eating something that you wish you hadn't (and that wasn't a healthy choice), you decide not to eat anything for the rest of the day so that you don't eat too many calories or too much sugar, and decide that the next day you will start over again. Doing this is very difficult on the body as you will be quite hungry by the time the evening rolls around. Instead of forgiving yourself, you are punishing yourself, and it will make it very hard not to reach for chips late at night when you are starving and feeling down.

- The fifth and final option is what you should do in this situation.

This option is the best for success and will make it the most likely to succeed long-term. If you fall off at lunch, let's say, because you are tired and in a rush, and you just grab something from a fast-food restaurant instead of going home for lunch or buying something at the grocery store to eat, this is how we will deal with it. Firstly, you will likely feel like you have failed and may feel quite down about making an unhealthy choice. Now instead of starving for the rest of the day or eating only lettuce for dinner, you will put this slip up at lunch behind you, and you will continue your day as if it never happened. You will eat a healthy dinner as you planned, and you will continue with the plan. You will not wait until tomorrow to begin again; you will continue as you would if you had made that healthy choice at lunch. The key to staying on track can bounce back. The people who can bounce back mentally are the ones who will be most likely to succeed. You will need to maintain a positive mental state and look forward to the rest of the day and the rest of the week in just the same way as you did before you had a slip-up. One bad meal out of the entire week will not ruin all of your progress, and recovering from emotional eating is largely a mental game. It is more mental than anything else, so we must not underestimate our mindset in our success or failure.

Using this type of thinking, you will set yourself up for success and not fall off your plan completely after one slip-up.

Tips For Success

One important way to ensure that these healthy choices stick for good is by changing certain lifestyle aspects. Doing this will reduce the chances of slipping up, which often happens when people eliminate them altogether. For example, you can change the way you approach the grocery store.

When you are entering the grocery store, you must change a few things about how you shop to set yourself up for success. These strategies are especially important when you are just beginning your intuitive eating practice. It will be challenging for you to enter the grocery store and avoid cravings and temptations.

The first thing to keep in mind when grocery shopping for a new diet is to enter with a list. By doing this, you are giving yourself a guide to follow, which will prevent you from picking up things that you are craving or things that you feel like eating at that moment.

One of the biggest things to keep in mind when beginning a new eating practice like intuitive eating is to avoid shopping when you are hungry. Doing this will make you reach for anything and everything that you see. By entering the grocery store when you are satiated or just eaten, you will stick to your list and avoid falling prey to temptations.

If you treat your grocery shopping experience like a treasure hunt, you will be able to cross things off of the list one at a time without venturing to the parts of the grocery store that will prove to be a challenge for you to resist. If you are making healthy eating choices, you will likely be spending most of your time at the perimeter of the grocery store. This location is where the whole, plant-based foods are located. By doing this and entering with a list, you will avoid the middle aisles where the processed, high-sugar temptation foods are all kept.

Having a plan is key when it comes to learning new habits and employing a new lifestyle. This plan can be as detailed as you wish, or it can simply come in the form of a general overview. I recommend you start with a more detailed plan in the beginning as you ease into things.

As everyone is different, you may be the type of person who likes lots of lists and plans, or you may be the type of person who doesn't, but for everyone, beginning with a plan and following it closely for the first little while is best. For example, this plan can include; what you will focus on each week, what you will reduce your intake of, and what you will try to achieve in terms of the mental work involved.

Once you have come up with a general plan for your new lifestyle and how you want it to look, you can begin laying out more specific plans.

Planning your meals will make it much easier for you when you get home from work or when you wake up tired in the morning and need to pack something for your lunch.

You can plan your meals out a week in advance, two weeks, or even a month if you wish. You can post this up on your fridge, and each day you will know exactly what you are eating, with no thinking required. This way, there won't be a chance for you to consider ordering a pizza or heating up some chicken fingers because you will already know exactly what you will make. By approaching your new style of eating in this way, you can make this transition easier on yourself and ensure success every step of the way.

Conclusion

Weight loss is much more than simply eating vegetables and going to the gym. This book taught you that weight loss involves much deeper concepts and much harder work than just this.

This book took a deep dive into various topics surrounding the psychology of body image, weight loss, and motivation. We looked at how you can control your internal self to accomplish anything and achieve your goals. This book aimed to equip you with the tools you need to control your life and change your body for the better. Through reading this book, I hope that you found some peace and a sense of compassion for yourself, as bringing about change is not an easy task.

We began by learning about some of the situations and causes that most often lead people to become overweight by looking at the connection between your mind and your physical body. We looked at some strategies for getting in touch with your emotions and feelings to determine what led you to where you currently are. We then learned about hypnosis and how it can help you make changes in your life. Now that you are equipped with various hypnosis techniques, you can begin practicing them in your daily life. Hypnosis is an invaluable tool for weight loss, and now that you have reached the end of this book, you are ready to take it into your own hands.

After addressing the psychological side of weight loss and body image, we learned about the science of weight loss, weight loss techniques, diets, and exercise. We looked at how you can plan around your lifestyle to ensure success. Finally, we looked at how to put everything we learned together in the form of a plan and how to deal with inevitable challenges or setbacks that you may face along the way.

It is important to remember that weight loss, a change of mind, or a change in rooted behaviors do not happen in one day or even in one week. The key to making any sort of change that will last in your life is consistency. You must be consistent in your hypnosis practice, diet, change of behaviors, and every component of your new lifestyle to see changes. If, for some reason, you slip up, remind yourself that you are not a failure and continue where you left off. This reminder will be the key to maintaining consistency and make changes in your life.

I hope that through reading this book, you have developed a deeper knowledge of how you can begin to change your life in much deeper ways than losing weight, but by also acknowledging and tackling the underlying causes of your unhappiness. By doing the hard work that this book helps you to realize, you can find lasting weight loss instead of a fluctuating number on the scale.

If you take one thing from this book, let it be the idea that you and your body must work as one. Do not fight with your mind or body, but instead work with it, and you will find harmony.

I wish you luck in your journey, and I hope that you continue to pursue lasting change.

Rapid Weight Loss Hypnosis for Women: Stop Emotional Hunger

Guided Hypnosis for Women Over 40. Want to Burn Fat Fast? With Meditation, Psychology, and Affirmation, You Will Finally Be Motivated to Do It. Increase Self-Esteem and Stop Premenopausal Nervous Hunger.

Gerald Paul Clifford

© Copyright 2020 by Gerald Paul Clifford. All right reserved.

The work contained herein has been produced with the intent to provide relevant knowledge and information on the topic on the topic described in the title for entertainment purposes only. While the author has gone to every extent to furnish up to date and true information, no claims can be made as to its accuracy or validity as the author has made no claims to be an expert on this topic. Notwithstanding, the reader is asked to do their own research and consult any subject matter experts they deem necessary to ensure the quality and accuracy of the material presented herein.

This statement is legally binding as deemed by the Committee of Publishers Association and the American Bar Association for the territory of the United States. Other jurisdictions may apply their own legal statutes. Any reproduction, transmission or copying of this material contained in this work without the express written consent of the copyright holder shall be deemed as a copyright violation as per the current legislation in force on the date of publishing and subsequent time thereafter. All additional works derived from this material may be claimed by the holder of this copyright.

The data, depictions, events, descriptions and all other information forthwith are considered to be true, fair and accurate unless the work is expressly described as a work of fiction. Regardless of the nature of this work, the Publisher is exempt from any responsibility of actions taken by the reader in conjunction with this work. The Publisher acknowledges that the reader acts of their own accord and releases the author and Publisher of any responsibility for the observance of tips, advice, counsel, strategies and techniques that may be offered in this volume.

Table of Contents

Introduction

Chapter 1: The Mind-Body Connection

What Is the Mind-Body Connection?

How Does the Mind-Body Connection Affect Your Life?

Common Mental Struggles That Manifest Themselves In The Body

    Childhood Trauma

    Covering Up Your Emotions

    Feeling Empty Or Feeling Bored

    Experiencing An Affection Deficiency

    Low Self-Esteem

    Low Mood

    Depression

    Anxiety

    Stress

    The Media

How These Struggles Can Lead People to Gain Weight

The Secret to Lasting Weight Loss

Chapter 2: Emotional Eating

What Is Emotional Eating?

What Is Binge Eating?

Why Does Emotional Eating Happen?

How to Tell if You Are Emotionally Eating

How to Read Your Hunger

The Science of Cravings and Food Addictions

Sugar Addictions: The Real Devil

How to Change Your Relationship With Food

Chapter 3: Addressing Your Current Mental State

What Are Core Wounds?

How to Address Your Core Wounds

    Journaling

    Self-Reflection

    Acknowledging Your Emotions

    Using Positive Self-Talk

What Is Positive Self-Talk?

How Can You Begin Using Positive Self-Talk?

Chapter 4: More Ways to Challenge Your Mind

How Self-Care Can Help

How to Practice Self-Care

Using Meditation

Meditation Techniques

What Is Mindful Eating?

The Benefits Of Mindful Eating

When and How to Use Mindful Eating

The Mindful Eating Technique

Chapter 5: Food-Related Changes to Begin Making

Making Good Food-Related Choices

How to Begin Making Good Choices Using Intuitive Eating

What Is Intuitive Eating?

The Benefits of Intuitive Eating

How to Make Intuitive Eating Part of Your Life

What Kind of Foods Should You Choose?

Electrolytes

Vitamin D

Chapter 6: Weight Loss

How to Achieve Weight Loss Without Using Diets

The Science of Weight Loss

How to Develop and Maintain a Healthy Diet Without Dieting

How to Shift Your Mind Toward Weight Loss

Chapter 7: Learning to Love Exercise

The Benefits of Exercise for Your Mental Health

How to Begin Using Exercise to Your Benefit

What Is Intuitive Movement?

Cardiovascular Exercise Versus Resistance Training

The Benefits of Other Kinds of Exercise

How Exercise Can Change Your Relationship With Your Body

The Importance of Sleep

Chapter 8: Using Affirmations

What Are Affirmations?

How Affirmations Will Benefit You

How to Use Affirmations

How to Come up With Affirmations of Your Own

Chapter 9: Hypnosis Techniques for Weight Loss

What Is Hypnosis?

The Benefits Of Hypnosis

The Different Levels Of Consciousness

   The Conscious Mind

   The Subconscious Mind

The 5 Levels Of Consciousness

How Can Hypnosis Help With Weight Loss?

Hypnosis For Cravings

Self-Hypnosis

Other Techniques

Visualization As A Form Of Self-Hypnosis

   What Is Visualization?

   The Benefits Of Visualization

   How To Use Visualization

Visualization for Creating a Plan of Action

Visualization for Achieving Goals That You Have Set Out for Yourself

Chapter 10: Motivation

What Is Motivation?

How To Find Motivation

How To Maintain Motivation

Self-Judgement And How To Overcome It

How to Make Your New Lifestyle a Habit

Tips For Success

Conclusion

Introduction

Welcome to my book, and thank you for choosing it! There are many other books on the market, and I am glad that you saw something in this one that made you choose it.

This book is a comprehensive guide for people who identify as women or those looking to support a woman in her weight loss journey. This book is for people who are eager to learn all that they can about weight loss, hypnosis, and how these two important concepts come together to help people achieve their goals! This book is for anyone who has struggled with weight loss or doesn't know where to begin weight loss. It doesn't matter what experience you bring to this book. It only matters that you have taken the first step by reading the first page!

This book will delve deeply into various topics surrounding the psychology of body image, weight loss, and motivation. We will look at how you can control your internal self to accomplish anything and achieve your goals. This book aims to equip you with the tools to control your life and body and make changes for the better. Through reading this book, I hope that you find some peace and a sense of compassion for yourself, as bringing about change is not an easy task.

We will begin by learning about some of the situations and causes that lead people to become overweight by looking at the connection between your mind and your physical body. We will look at some strategies for getting in touch with your emotions and feelings to self-evaluate and determine what led you to where you are currently. This book's philosophy involves looking deep within to find the root causes and deal with the issues once and for all, instead of finding band-aid solutions like most books of this sort.

We will then look at hypnosis and how it can help you make changes in your life through various hypnosis practices. We will look at hypnosis and how it impacts the mind-body connection, and the science behind why it has been proven to work.

We will examine how hypnosis can be useful for weight loss and how you can set yourself up for success, especially if you have been attempting to lose weight unsuccessfully for some time. We will also look at visualization to increase the chances of success and help you with any goals you have set for yourself in your life.

Our next topic will be Emotional Eating, which is rarely discussed, but that cannot be left out of the narrative. By examining your eating patterns, you can determine whether you are an emotional eater, which will help you to better understand how to approach your weight loss plan.

After addressing the psychological side of weight loss and body image, we will delve more into the science of weight loss, weight loss techniques, diets, and exercise. We will look at how you can plan for yourself to work with your lifestyle to ensure success. Finally, we will look at how to put everything we have discussed together in the form of a plan and deal with setbacks or challenges that you will likely face along the way.

In the first chapter of this book, we will discuss the mind-body connection and how this may be presenting itself in your life. Be prepared for some self-reflection and realization, which is the first step in making any changes in one's life.

This book will delve into various topics surrounding weight loss and hypnosis, including but not limited to the following;

- The mind-body connection and how this plays a crucial role in your weight loss journey

- How to use affirmations and self-hypnosis to achieve your goals of lasting weight loss

- How to use meditation to combat food cravings and overcome food addictions (we all have them!)

- How to break free from the reigns of sugar cravings and sugar dependence

- How to lose weight FOR GOOD without the use of diets that make you feel defeated

- How to use the technique of mindful eating

- Essential techniques and strategies for using self-hypnosis

- Tips and tricks for finding and maintaining motivation to stick to your plan

- How to overcome binge eating and how to change your relationship with food

Without further ado, let's begin, but before moving onto the first chapter of this book, I want to give a brief disclaimer;

This book is not supposed to replace medical advice. It is not responsible for the actions or the results of the reader. Please seek out the advice of a doctor before starting any health program. The author is not a medical doctor, and the information in this book is meant only to supplement your health decisions and actions, not dictate them. Scientists are still researching the wonders of Autophagy at this very moment, even as I write this book. Please enjoy the information provided but also be wise in consuming it.

Now, let's get to the good stuff!

Chapter 1: The Mind-Body Connection

In this chapter, I will begin the book by talking about something called the *mind-body connection*. This idea may seem self-explanatory, but we will be delving into some pretty deep territory, so I will begin with the basics, and we will move on from there.

What Is the Mind-Body Connection?

This chapter talks about the *mind-body connection*, which is the term used to describe a concept that states that a person's internal or mental state (their thoughts, feelings, beliefs, etc.) can lead to physical, biological events, changes, or repercussions in the body.

How Does the Mind-Body Connection Affect Your Life?

You may be wondering how these two seemingly unrelated things (the inner world and the outer body) can be considered related. Over time, your body learns that eating certain foods (like those containing processed sugars or salts such as fast food and quick pastries) makes the body feel rewarded, positive and happy for some time after these foods are ingested.

When you feel sad or worried, your body feels this and looks for ways to remedy these negative feelings. Your brain then connects the mind's feelings with the reward that it knows that it can get from eating certain foods. As a result, eating these foods will turn its inner state from negative to positive and make it feel better.

As this process happens in your mind's background without you being aware of it, you then consciously feel a craving for those foods (like sugary snacks or salty fast-food meals) as a result. You may not even be aware of why you are craving them, as it all happens so fast in the subconscious mind. If you decide to give in to this craving and eat something like a microwave pizza snack, your body will feel rewarded and happy for a brief period. This process reinforces the concept believed by your brain that craving food to make itself feel better emotionally has worked.

If you feel down and guilty that you ate something unhealthy, your brain will again try and remedy these negative emotions by craving food. This process is how a cycle of emotional eating can then begin without you being any the wiser.

Because scientists and psychiatrists come to understand this process in the brain and the body, they know that the mind and the body are inextricably connected. Those food cravings or even being overweight can often indicate emotional deficiencies in emotional struggles.

For this reason, it is important to address the underlying issues when trying to lose weight or stop the cycle of emotional eating. By dealing with the root causes of the problem, you can stop it from reoccurring. If you simply try to follow a crash diet for some time without looking deep within to find the causes of the struggles you are having, the chances of falling back into emotional eating are very high. Therefore, it is necessary to address the root causes to end emotional eating once and for all.

Common Mental Struggles That Manifest Themselves In The Body

Now that you understand how a person's internal environment can lead them to fall into a cycle of emotional eating or seek food as comfort and eventually become overweight, we will look at some of the factors that lead people to develop a tumultuous internal environment.

Several types of emotional deficiencies or causes can lead a person to develop disordered eating, resulting in weight gain over time. We will explore some of these factors in detail in hopes that you will recognize some of the reasons why you may experience struggles with eating or with weight loss.

Childhood Trauma

The first example of an emotional deficiency that we will examine is more of an umbrella for various emotional deficiencies. This umbrella term is Childhood Causes. If you think back on your childhood, think about how your relationship with food was cultivated. Maybe you were taught that when you behaved, you received food as a reward. Maybe when you were feeling down, you were given food to cheer you up. Maybe you turned to food when you were experiencing negative events that happened during your childhood.

Another cause could be the relationship you had with your parents or the relationship to food modeled for you in your formative years. Maybe you grew up in an emotionally abusive home, and food was the only comfort you had. These reasons are completely valid, which was the only way you knew how to deal with problems when you were a child. The positive thing is that you can take control of your life and make lasting changes for the better now that you are an adult.

Any of these experiences could cause someone to suffer from emotional eating in their adulthood, as it had become something learned from an early age. This type of emotional deficiency is quite difficult to break as it has likely been a habit for many, many years, but it is possible.

When we are children, we learn habits and make associations without knowing it that we often carry into our later lives. While this is no fault of yours, recognizing it as a potential issue is important to make changes.

Covering Up Your Emotions

Another emotional deficiency that can manifest itself in emotional eating and food cravings is the effort to cover up our emotions. Sometimes we would rather distract ourselves and cover up our emotions than to feel them or to face them head-on. In this case, our brain may make us feel hungry to distract us with the act of eating food. When we have a quiet minute where these feelings or thoughts pop into our minds, we can cover them up by deciding to prepare food and eat and convince ourselves that we are "too busy" to acknowledge our feelings because we have to deal with our hunger. The fact that it is a hunger that arises in this scenario makes it very difficult to ignore and very easy to deem as a necessary distraction. After all, we do need to eat to survive. This necessity can be a problem, though, if we do not require nourishment and we are telling ourselves that this is why we cannot deal with our demons or our emotions. If there is something that you think you may be avoiding dealing with or thinking about, or if you tend to be very uncomfortable with feelings of unrest, you may be experiencing this type of emotional eating.

Feeling Empty Or Feeling Bored

When we feel bored, we often decide to eat or decide that we are hungry. This hunger occupies our mind and our time and makes us feel less bored and even feel positive and happy. We also may eat when we are feeling empty. When we feel empty, the food will quite literally be ingested to fill a void. Still, as we know, the food will not fill a void that is emotional in sort, and this will lead to an unhealthy cycle of trying to fill ourselves emotionally with something that will never actually work. This process will lead us to become disappointed every time and continue trying to fill this void with material things like food or purchases. This compulsion can also be caused because of a general feeling of dissatisfaction with life and lack of something in your life. Looking deeper into this the next time you feel those cravings will be difficult but will help you greatly in the long term as you will then be able to identify the source of your feelings of emptiness and begin to fill these voids in ways that will be much more effective.

Experiencing An Affection Deficiency

Another emotional deficiency that could manifest itself as food cravings is an affection deficiency. This type of deficiency can be feelings of loneliness, feelings of a lack of love, or feelings of being undesired. Suppose a person has been without an intimate relationship or has recently gone through a breakup, or has not experienced physical intimacy in quite some time. In that case, they may be experiencing an affection deficiency. This type of emotional deficiency will often manifest itself in food cravings. We will try to gain comfort and positivity from the good tasting, drug-like (as we talked about in chapter one) foods they crave.

Low Self-Esteem

Another emotional deficiency that may be indicated by food cravings is a low level of self-esteem. Low self-esteem can cause people to feel down, unlovable, inadequate, and overall negative and sad. This feeling can make a person feel like eating foods they enjoy will make them feel better, even for a mere few moments. Low self-esteem is an emotional deficiency that is difficult to deal with, as it affects every area of a person's life, such as their love life, social life, career life, etc. Sometimes, people have reported feeling like food was always there for them and never left them. While this is true, they will often be left feeling even emptier and lower about themselves after giving into cravings.

Low Mood

A general low mood can cause emotional eating. While the problem of emotional eating is something that is occurring multiple times per week, and we all have general low moods or bad days, if this makes you crave food and especially food of an unhealthy sort, this could become emotional eating. When we feel down or are having a bad day, we want to eat food to make ourselves feel better; this is emotional eating. Some people will want a drink at the end of a bad day. If this happens every once in a while, it is not necessarily a problem with emotional eating. The more often it happens, the more often it is emotional eating. Further, we do not have to give in to the cravings to be considered emotional eating. Experiencing the cravings often and in tandem with negative feelings in the first place is what constitutes emotional eating.

Depression

Suffering from depression also can lead to emotional eating. Depression is a constant low mood for months on end, and this low mood can cause a person to turn to food for comfort and a lift in spirit. This lifting feeling can then become emotional eating in addition to and because of depression.

Anxiety

Having anxiety can lead to emotional eating, as well. There are several types of anxiety, and whether it is general anxiety (constant levels of anxiety), situational anxiety (triggered by a situation or scenario) can lead to emotional eating. You have likely heard of the term *comfort food* to describe certain foods and dishes. The reason for this is because they are usually foods rich in carbohydrates, fats, and heavy. These foods bring people a sense of comfort. These foods are often turned to when people suffering from anxiety are emotionally eating because they temporarily ease their anxiety and make them feel calmer and more at ease. This calming effect only lasts for a short period; however, before their anxiety usually gears up again.

Stress

Stress eating is probably the most common form of emotional eating. While this does not become an issue for everyone experiencing stress, it is a problem for people who consistently turn to food to ease their stress. Some people are always under stress, and they will constantly be looking for ways to ease their stress. Food is one of these ways that people use to make themselves feel better and to take their minds off of their stress. As with all of the other examples we have seen above, this is not a lasting resolution, and it becomes a cycle. Similar to the cycle that I discussed above, the same can be used for stress. In the case of stress, instead of a negative emotion making you feel down, stress eating can make you feel more stressed, as you can begin to feel like you have done something you shouldn't have done, which causes you to stress, and the stress eating cycle ensues.

The Media

The constant exposure to media that we experience on a day to day basis can lead to a negative internal environment over time. If you are constantly seeing photos of people who make you feel inadequate, or people to whom you are comparing yourself, you can begin to believe that you are not good enough or that you will never measure up. These thoughts can be damaging and can lead a person to turn to food for comfort. This coping mechanism can lead them to feel worse about themselves afterward, leading to even more emotional eating.

How These Struggles Can Lead People to Gain Weight

As we have seen so far in this chapter, there are various reasons why people may develop a negative internal environment in terms of their thoughts, feelings, and attitudes. Over time, this can lead to changes in a person's physical body, such as weight gain. These changes are clear evidence of the mind-body connection at work. This emotional turmoil could be due to any of the reasons I previously mentioned, such as stress or childhood trauma, and it can begin to cause a person to seek food as a means of comfort. If this is done over a prolonged period, it can lead a person to gain weight steadily until they reach a dangerous level of obesity. Then, because they may begin to feel bad about their physical appearance, they may turn to food to comfort them for their body's negative thoughts and feelings.

This feeling can lead a person to gain weight if these struggles lead to *binge eating*. Binge eating is a disorder that can be seen along with emotional eating much of the time. Binge eating disorder is when a person eats much more than a regular amount of food on a single occasion or sitting, and they feel unable to control themselves or stop themselves. This effect could also be defined as a compulsion to overeat. It has to happen at least two times per week for longer than six months consecutively to be considered a disorder. Binge eating and overeating may appear to be the same, though they are sometimes seen as individual disorders. Overeating is when a person eats more than they require to sustain life. This overeating occurs when they consume much more than they need in a day or a single sitting.

Overeating does not necessarily become binge eating, but it certainly can. Overeating is a general term used to describe the eating disorders that we just defined-Emotional Eating and Binge Eating. Thus, overeating could involve binge eating, food addiction, or other food-related disorders.

Throughout the rest of this book, we will be examining ways to combat this (including using hypnosis) to restore both physical health and a positive mental state to ultimately break the cycle of emotional eating and help you lose weight for good!

The Secret to Lasting Weight Loss

Recognizing the food-related struggles you face will also help you to have a better relationship with your body. Instead of seeing it as; something that you dislike the shape of, something that causes you to feel hungry when you do not need to eat, something that makes you feel guilty when you eat, and something that has disordered eating processes, you can begin to love and care for your body by providing it with nourishment, clean energy, and adequate hydration.

Viewing your body as something to care for (as it is the thing that carries you around all day and houses your most important parts) will allow you to shift your view of yourself and your body to begin seeing it in a more positive light. You can begin to see your body as something you can work together with instead of something you work against.

Recognizing your struggles will also help you to have a better relationship with your mind. Understanding how your mind works will help you to better take care of it. You will be able to recognize your feelings and what they could be caused by, and then treat them in a way that will help it to feel better. Bettering your relationship with food and your body will also improve your relationship with your mind. This relationship will improve because you will begin to feed it what it needs, which will, in turn, lead to better cognitive functioning, control over impulses (like impulses to give in to cravings), and decision-making. This effect will help overall in your relationships with your food, your body, and your mind.

As you can see, dealing with the mind and its struggles is the secret to lasting weight loss and happy life overall. Throughout this book, we will address the mental struggles and help you to break free from them. It will not be an easy process, but it will be well worth it.

Be gentle with yourself throughout this process, as it will be uncomfortable at times and will require strength. This book will help you through it, as you are not alone. I hope that this book also reminds you that many other people are suffering from the same type of food-related disorders as you are and that you are not alone in that either. This book will take a step-by-step approach, which will make for the highest chance of recovery. If at any time you need to take a break to think about the information you have learned, feel free to do so, but make sure you come back to this book quite soon after. Going through this recovery process can be a lot, but it will be possible with the right support.

You have already taken the first step in recovery, which is acknowledging that you have an issue. For that, I congratulate you!

Chapter 2: Emotional Eating

Before we begin looking at the concrete methods that you can use to begin losing weight and breaking free from your mental struggles, we will learn a little more about something called *emotional eating*. I briefly touched on this in the previous chapter, but here we will delve deeper into it before moving on.

What Is Emotional Eating?

As we discussed in the previous chapter, emotional eating occurs when a person suffering from emotional deficiencies of some sort (including a lack of affection, lack of connection, stress, depression, anxiety, or feelings like sadness and anger) eats as a means of gaining comfort from the food they are eating.

Many people find comfort in food. When people experience negative feelings and turn to food consumption to reduce their pain or feel better, this is called emotional eating. Some people do this on occasion, like after a breakup or after a bad fight, but when this occurs at least a few times a week, it negatively impacts one's life. At this point, it becomes an issue that needs to be addressed. Thank you for taking the time to work on yourself in this way, and I am here with you at each step.

What Is Binge Eating?

Another form of disordered eating that is often seen, along with emotional eating, is *binge eating*. I defined this term in the previous chapter, but we will revisit it here briefly.

Binge eating disorder is when a person eats much more than a regular amount of food on a single occasion or sitting, and they feel unable to control themselves or stop themselves. This person could also be experiencing a compulsion to overeat.

To be considered a "Binge Eating Disorder," it must happen at least two times per week for longer than six months consecutively. If this is not the case, it can still negatively affect a person's life, but it would not be considered a Binge Eating Disorder diagnosis.

Why Does Emotional Eating Happen?

Emotional eating occurs because eating foods that we enjoy makes us feel rewarded on our brains' emotional and physiological levels.

People binge eat for a very similar reason to the reason why people experience emotional eating. This reason is that eating foods that we enjoy in terms of taste, smell, texture, etc., makes us feel rewarded on our brains' emotional and physiological level.

Throughout this chapter, we will look more in-depth at these eating disorders to give you more information about why they occur and what could cause them.

How to Tell if You Are Emotionally Eating

Because scientists and psychiatrists understand the brain's chemical reward process when a person emotionally eats, they know that there are different types of food cravings. There are food cravings that indicate emotional deficiencies and the types of cravings that pregnant women experience. Because they understand the science behind it, researchers have come up with ways to tell if some type of emotional deficiency causes a craving.

This method begins by determining the foods that a person craves and when they crave them. For example, if every time someone has a stressful situation, they feel like eating a pizza, or if a person who is depressed tends to eat a lot of chocolate, this could indicate emotional eating. As you know by now, emotional eating and bulimia are closely related, and emotional eating can lead to bulimia over time.

If you crave fruit like a watermelon on a hot day, you are likely just dehydrated, and your body is trying to get water from a water-filled fruit that it knows will make it more hydrated. Examining situations like this has led scientists and psychiatrists to explore eating disorders in more depth and determine what types of emotional deficiencies can manifest themselves through food cravings or disordered eating in this way.

Recognizing your triggers is important because this will allow you to notice when you may be feeling emotional hunger and when you are feeling actual hunger. If you become hungry, you can look back on your day or the last hour and determine if any of your triggers were present. If they were, you would determine that you are likely experiencing emotional hunger, and you can take the appropriate steps instead of giving in to the cravings blindly.

There are many different emotional causes for the cravings we experience. There may be others than those listed in the previous chapter, and these are all valid. A person's emotional eating experience is unique and personal and could be caused by many things. You may also experience a combination of emotional deficiencies or one of those listed in addition to others. Many of these can overlap, such as anxiety and depression, often seen together in a single person. The level of these emotional deficiencies that you experience could indicate the level of emotional eating you struggle with. Whatever experiences or struggles you are dealing with, there is the hope of recovery, and this is what the rest of this book will focus on.

In the next chapter, we will learn several ways to determine your mental state so that you can begin to combat emotional eating.

How to Read Your Hunger

Now that you understand emotional eating, we will look at the different types of hunger and how you can tell them apart. This section will help you distinguish when you are hungry and when you may turn to food to soothe your emotional state.

Real hunger is when our body needs nutrients or energy and lets us know that we should soon replenish our energy. This feeling happens when it has been a few hours since our last meal when we wake up in the morning, or after a lot of strenuous activity like a long hike. Our body uses hunger to signal to us that it needs more energy and that if it doesn't get it soon, it will begin to use our stored energy as fuel. While there is nothing wrong with our body using its stored fuel, it can be used as a sign that we should eat shortly to replenish these stores.

Perceived hunger is when we think we are hungry, but our body doesn't require any more energy or the stores to be replenished. This kind of hunger can happen for several reasons, including an emotional deficiency, a negative mental state, or the occurrence of a psychological trigger.

The Science of Cravings and Food Addictions

We may often see ingredients on the packages of foods we eat, but we aren't sure of exactly what they are, just that they taste good. This section will take a deeper look at them and what they do to your brain.

Casein is a heavily processed ingredient that is derived from milk. It is processed a few times over and eventually creates concentrated milk solids. These milk solids- called Casein are then added into foods like cheese, french fries, milkshakes, and other fast and convenient packaged or fast-foods that contain dairy or dairy products (such as pastries and salad dressings). Casein has been compared to nicotine in its addictive properties. It is often seen in cheese, and this is why there is increasing evidence that people can become, and many are already addicted to cheese. The reason for this is during digestion. When cheese and other foods that contain Casein are digested, it is broken down, and one of the compounds that it breaks down into is a compound that is strikingly similar to opioids. This highly addictive substance is in pain killers.

High fructose corn syrup is surely an ingredient you have heard of before or at least one you have seen on the packaging of your favorite snacks or quick foods. While this is derived from real corn, after it is finished being processed, there is nothing corn-like about it. High fructose corn syrup is essentially the same thing as refined sugar when all is said and done. It is used as a sweetener in foods like soda, cereal, and other sweet and quick foods. This ingredient is often seen because it is much cheaper than using sugar and is much easier to work with.

High Fructose Corn Syrup is another common food additive that is highly addictive. This substance is similar to cocaine in its addictive properties.

MSG stands for Monosodium Glutamate, which sounds a lot like a chemical you may have encountered in science class in college. MSG is added to foods to give them a delicious flavor. It is essentially a very concentrated form of salt. What this does (in foods such as fast-food, packaged convenience foods, and buffet-style food) is that it gives it that wonderfully salty and fatty flavor that makes us keep coming back for more. Companies put this in food because it comes at an extremely low cost, and the flavor it brings covers up the artificial flavors of all of the other cheap ingredients used to make these foods. MSG has been known to block our natural appetite suppressant, which normally kicks in when we have had enough to eat. For this reason, when we are eating foods containing MSG, we do not recognize when we are satiated, and we continue to eat until we are stuffed because it tastes so great.

Sugar Addictions: The Real Devil

We will now look more closely at sugar and how it affects our bodies and our minds. Sugar is the worst culprit of all of these food additives. Sugar is responsible for this because it is so hard to avoid! Sugar is found in everything we eat that we can buy from a restaurant or a store. There are many sugar forms and so many names disguised as in the ingredients list on food packaging. One food may contain 70 percent sugar, but on the label, it may look as if this is not true because the different types of sugar have all been separated to trick us into thinking this is not the case. When it comes to avoiding sugar, it takes diligence and a keen eye for detail.

We already discussed one form of sugar, High Fructose Corn Syrup. This sugar type is cheap and easy to get your hands on, so it is added to virtually everything packaged that we can ingest. It is added because it gives even salty foods that tasty flavor balance.

As we discussed previously in this chapter, the chemicals found in food act in our brains very similar to how highly addictive drugs act. Sugar itself acts in a specific way that makes it so difficult to avoid. Sugar affects what is called the *Limbic System*. The limbic system is a group of structures in the brain that have to do with our emotions and memory. This system includes the regulation of our emotions and forming memories, which contributes to our learning.

For this reason, when we eat something very sugary, the chemicals that make up the sugars can affect our emotions. When this happens, it makes us feel emotions like happiness and satisfaction. Then, because eating certain foods makes us feel like this, we form a memory of this, and in turn, we learn that eating these specific foods gives us positive emotions. These emotions make us keep coming back for more.

So, when we eat something that contains both sugars and Casein, for example, we will get action on our limbic system and our reward system in the brain. Therefore, foods that give us both a feeling of reward and a surge of positive emotion are the most difficult to resist and the first ones we turn to when we want comfort in the form of food because we know they will make us feel good. And they always do, as these chemical reactions in the brain occur each time. We may not even realize this, as it becomes second nature to us. We may not recognize the positive feelings we get after we eat something that comforts us, but we know we keep craving it for some reason. If this has ever happened to you, you now know why this is. After learning about these things, pay attention to your cravings and see if this may be the explanation for why you have them. Pay attention also to the times that these cravings occur. Did you just receive some bad news? Was it on a rainy day when you were feeling especially down? Hold onto this information as we will revisit it shortly. Later on, in this book, we will also be discussing several ways to overcome these challenges to break the cycles of emotional eating and overeating.

How to Change Your Relationship With Food

The key to solving the food-related struggles that you face is to address your core wounds. Understanding how your mind works will help you to better take care of it. You will be able to recognize your feelings and how they could have come about, and then treat them in a way that will help it to feel better. Bettering your relationship with food and your body will also improve your relationship with your mind. This relationship will then allow you to begin to feed it what it needs, which will, in turn, lead to better cognitive functioning, control over impulses, and decision-making. This better functioning will help overall your relationship with your food, body, and mind.

In the next chapter, we will take a deeper look into these core wounds, and I will begin teaching you strategies to deal with them. Through the next chapter and those that follow, we will begin learning how to deal with emotional eating.

Chapter 3: Addressing Your Current Mental State

In this chapter, we will look at how you can begin to tackle your mind to make positive changes for your body and break free from your eating disorder once and for all.

We will begin by looking at core wounds before learning how to deal with them and ultimately change your relationship with food.

What Are Core Wounds?

As discussed in the previous chapter, there are several types of emotional deficiencies indicated by disordered eating. Once you have determined which of these emotional deficiencies (or which combination of them) are present in your life, you can begin to look at them in a little more detail. By doing so, you will come upon your core wounds. A core wound is something that you believe to be true about yourself or your life, and it is something that likely came about as a result of a coping mechanism you developed to deal with childhood. For example, this could be something like; the feeling of not being enough, the belief that you are unlovable, or the belief that you are stupid.

How to Address Your Core Wounds

By understanding and addressing your core wounds, you will be able to change your behaviors because of the intricate relationship that exists between your thoughts, your emotions, and your behaviors. By addressing your thoughts and emotions, you will change your behaviors and free yourself from eating disordered. You may be wondering how you can begin to address your core wounds, as it can be difficult to know where to begin.

The first step is learning to control and change your thoughts, which, in turn, leads to changes in your behavior. By taking control of your thoughts and beliefs, they don't have the opportunity to manifest into unhealthy behaviors such as overeating, turning to food for comfort, or any other unhealthy coping mechanisms that you have developed throughout your life.

Becoming aware of your thoughts is the most crucial step in this entire guide, as everything else will fail without it. Paying attention to your thoughts will help you identify what thoughts are going through your mind during an intense emotional moment. By looking deep within, to get in touch with your deepest feelings, you will be more likely to succeed in weight loss and overall lifestyle improvement.

Journaling

One great example of how to put this into practice is through the use of journaling. Journaling can help in a process such as this because it can help you organize your thoughts and feelings and visually see what is working and what isn't working for you. While we can give tips and examples, every person is different, so to find exactly what works for you, you will have to try different things and see which techniques help you personally the most and in the best way. Journaling can be about anything like how you feel since beginning a new program, how you feel physically since changing your diet, how you feel emotionally now that you are not reaching for food to comfort your emotions and anything along these lines.

Self-Reflection

Doing some serious and deep self-reflection is not an easy process but a necessary one for healing yourself and changing your habits that are so ingrained. Looking deep within and asking yourself the proper questions will help you take the first step, acknowledging the issues and finding their sources. Finding the sources will tell you exactly what you need to face and deal with to achieve a lasting change of this new intuitive eating lifestyle.

If changing your life is a distraction from the underlying issues, the change will not be lasting. These issues will rise to the surface again eventually, and they will manifest themselves in strong cravings. I want you to permanently change your life, and to do this; we will begin with some deep self-reflection. You will get out of this workbook what you put in, so take your time as you go through this chapter and try to get in touch with the deeper parts of yourself.

We will begin the self-reflection with some questions to ask yourself to get into a self-examination mindset. Complete this workbook, and you will be well on your way to dealing with your emotions, as you will have a better idea of what these emotions are.

1. Do I feel like I struggle with emotional eating?

Yes ____ No ____

2. Do I wish to find out the underlying causes of my emotional eating?

Yes ____ No ____

3. Do I feel like it is time for a lifestyle change in terms of my eating habits?

Yes ____ No ____

The first question you will ask yourself is a rather obvious one, but this will make it easy for you to get a start on your self-examination.

8. Have I been diagnosed with mood-related disorders (such as depression, bipolar disorder, or anxiety)?

Yes ____ No____

If your answer is yes, you skip section 2. If you answered No and you are unsure if you suffer from one of these, complete section 2.

9. Do I have long periods of low mood or an anxious state?

Yes ____ No ____

10. Have I been feeling this way for the last 3 to 6 months?

Yes ____ No ____

11. Do I often feel disconnected from my life?

Yes ____ No ____

12. Do I often feel nervous and worried about worst-case scenarios?

Yes ____ No ____

13. Do I often catastrophize in my head when thinking about things that are to come?

Yes ____ No ____

14. Do I often feel drastic swings between very high moods (like happy, excited, and motivated) and very low moods (sad, down, hopeless)

Yes ____ No ____

If you answered mostly Yes to the questions above, you might suffer from a mood-related disorder. While this questionnaire is not conclusive and is not sanctioned by a doctor or a medical professional, this could give you a bit of direction regarding your mood, emotions, and the causes of your emotional eating. Knowing that the cause could be something like depression, anxiety, or another mood disorder can give you some clarity on your mental state. If you think this could be the case, consider visiting your doctor to discuss this further with someone who is especially knowledgeable in these areas.

Acknowledging Your Emotions

It is very important to notice and address your feelings, as they can tell you many important things.

Pay attention to your thoughts, and whenever you feel a negative emotion, work backward. Try to figure out what thoughts were just on your mind before you felt negative emotions. Emotions that you should be looking out for are stress, anxiety, self-loathing, sadness, demotivation, anger, and frustration. These emotions are the ones that typically cause a person to choose instant gratification.

Just like how you will be paying attention to the thoughts that occurred before feeling a negative emotion, pay attention to the thoughts that occurred before feeling a positive emotion. By identifying what those thoughts were, you will begin to learn what types of thoughts bring positive emotions. Typically, when a person feels positive emotions, it creates more motivation and inspiration to reach goals.

One great way to begin feeling your emotions is by self-reflecting and noticing when they are causing you struggles related to food. Below are some more specific questions that will help prompt you to look at your emotions more deeply.

- Emotional Triggers

What are some triggers related to your emotions or specific emotions that make you seek comfort in the form of food? For example: When I feel scared, I begin to crave sweets.

- Additional Triggers

Are there any other triggers that you experience that cause your emotional deficiencies to flare up? For example: When I go to school, I feel lonely.

Recognizing your triggers is important because this will allow you to notice when you may be feeling emotional hunger and when you are feeling actual hunger. If you become hungry, you can look back on your day or the last hour and determine if any of your triggers were present. If they were, you would be able to determine that you are likely experiencing emotional hunger, and you can take the appropriate steps instead of giving in to the cravings blindly. These triggers tie into emotional eating because when you experience a trigger that causes one of your emotional deficiencies to become more apparent to you (or to act up), you are most likely to turn to food as a means of comfort and as a way to self-soothe. Recognizing what these triggers are will help you to recognize when to intervene in your normal cognitive processes such as "I am hungry" "I am going to eat a cookie." Instead of this normal process that would occur after a situation or an emotion triggers your feelings of loneliness, for example, you will know to intervene, and instead, it will go something like this; "I am hungry," "Am I hungry or feeling an emotional need?", "A trigger just occurred, so I am going to call a friend and talk instead of eating what I crave."

Using Positive Self-Talk

Once you have addressed your emotions and your core wounds, you can begin to intervene and change them to result in healthier behaviors. You will do this using positive self-talk. Adopting helpful thought processes fosters better emotions overall, which leads to more productive behaviors.

When people have developed unhelpful thinking processes, it is hard to make decisions that will benefit their future selves because their thoughts create negative emotions that drive away motivation. This situation is where something called *positive self-talk* can come in. Positive self-talk can be instrumental in helping you to recover from disordered eating.

What Is Positive Self-Talk?

Their inner critic controls many people's minds. The inner critic shares words with you, such as "You should just give up" Or "What makes you think you'll succeed?" which is rooted in the opposite of positive self-talk- Negative self-talk!

Instead of creating an open space that allows for mistakes, growth, and development, your inner critic causes you to question your worth. This questioning makes it difficult for you to have the positive, growth mindset needed to complete tasks and go after things that may be difficult to achieve. In this case, helping your mind begin using positive self-talk will help you recover for the long-term.

How Can You Begin Using Positive Self-Talk?

Below are several ways that you can begin to use positive self-talk. Over time, your mind will get used to thinking in this way, and you will find it much easier to do.

6. Remind yourself

Bad habits are built through many years, and no amount of willpower can undo a lifetime of bad habits, such as a strong inner critic that uses negative self-talk. By rewiring your brain to minimize the amount of negativity you feel in the first place, you will eventually get used to filling your mind with positive thoughts instead of negative ones.

7. Stop the automatic process of negativity.

Often, if the person had just paid attention to their thought process, they would be able to catch themselves before their mind automatically spiraled to a place of complete demotivation. By catching yourself before you get there, you can prevent yourself from falling into your negative thought patterns, limiting you and holding you back.

8. Find positive influences

Surrounding yourself with people that can encourage you and foster positivity will also change your inner-critic's opinion. Often, hearing positive compliments from other people hold a heavier weight in the eyes of your inner-critic compared to you telling your inner-critic the same thing. Try spending time with people who support your goals and the changes you are looking to make in your life. It will make your journey a little bit easier.

9. Limit Negative Influences

By limiting your life's negative influences, you are making a statement to yourself that you place importance on preserving your mental health. When you remove negative influences and limit your exposure to things or people that make you feel negative, you prioritize yourself, which is a great way to practice self-care.

10. Practice a gratitude exercise

This exercise is a great exercise to remind yourself of everything you love and appreciate yourself and your life. Take time to write down all of the things that you love about yourself and your life. Doing this will remind you of all of the positivity surrounding you and will serve to uplift you.

Chapter 4: More Ways to Challenge Your Mind

In this chapter, we will look at how you can begin to tackle your mind to make positive changes for your body and break free from your eating disorder once and for all.

How Self-Care Can Help

Self-Care is the method by which you will begin to love and to take care of your body. Self-care includes both your physical and your mental health. When you begin to take care of yourself physically and mentally, you will begin to see many changes come about, namely an increase in positive feelings and a decrease in negative ones.

How to Practice Self-Care

There are numerous ways that you can practice self-care, and these ways can be different for everyone. In this section, I will outline some ways to practice self-care to begin feeling more positive about yourself and your body and begin changing your internal environment around you.

- You Are Worthy

This exercise is a great exercise to remind yourself of everything you love and appreciate yourself and your life. Take time to write down all of the things that you love about yourself and your life. Doing this will remind you of all of the positivity surrounding you and will serve to uplift you.

- Limit Negative Influences

By limiting your life's negative influences, you are making a statement to yourself that you place importance on preserving your mental health. When you remove negative influences and limit your exposure to things or people that make you feel negative, you prioritize yourself, which is a great way to practice self-care.

Included here are also the negative influences that you have over yourself. Limiting beliefs and negative self-talk, and a negative body image can lead a person to feel terrible about themselves, often to the point of feeling like they hate themselves. As I mentioned earlier, to make lasting changes, we will work on loving ourselves instead of hating ourselves. By positively seeing your body, you will begin to make choices with your body's health in mind because of all of the things it allows you to do. This process will lead to lasting, positive changes for your physical and mental health.

- Support System

Finding a positive and uplifting support system helps improve and preserve your mental health. This system can be one person or a group of people. It can include family or friends or acquaintances, as long as they support you in your journey and help you to feel positive about your life and yourself in general. Some examples of places you can find a support system include Facebook groups, support groups, weight loss support groups, and books. Not only will a support system help you to move toward positivity, but when you begin to make changes in your life, your support system will help by supporting you in maintaining these changes.

- Journaling

Another journaling exercise you can do to change your limiting beliefs is writing down all of the limiting beliefs you think you possess. Then, try to think of and write down where you think they came from. For example, try to think of where you learned to think this way or where this was modeled for you. Having this information written down in front of you can help you to begin changing them, as awareness is the first step to change.

- Notice And Challenge Your Inner Critic

The negative self-talk that many people experience comes from something called their *inner critic*. Your inner critic lives in a black and white world, a world with very little room for the grey area, and where failure is the worst possible outcome of every scenario. Your inner critic shares words with you, such as, "You should just give up" Or "What makes you think you'll succeed?" Instead of creating an open space that allows for mistakes, growth, and development, your inner critic causes you to question your worth. These thoughts make it difficult for you to have the positive, growth mindset needed to complete tasks and go after things that may be difficult to achieve. For some people, their inner critic is reminiscent of a voice from their past- it could be their mother, father, or person who bullied them. For others, it could simply be their voice criticizing them for everything they do. Sometimes, if a person makes an offhand comment at you, this could lead you to absorb it so deeply that the words they said become a part of your identity.

Awareness is the first step that needs to be taken to recognize your inner-critic and reshape it into something less critical and more supportive. Try to pay attention the next time you are feeling distracted, numb, or anxious. Try to identify whose voice is the voice of your inner critic. Try to find the situation where your inner critic awakens. Allows yourself to dig deep and identify the most vulnerable feelings during situations where your inner critic is awake. These feelings or these situations are likely what your inner critic is trying to protect you from feeling. However, by protecting you, they are holding you back from meeting your full potential.

Using Meditation

Simply put, meditation is a practice where a person uses a technique, like mindfulness - to focus their thoughts and mind on an activity, thought, or object to train their awareness and attention. The goal of this is to help the person achieve clear-headedness and an emotionally calm and stable state.

The simplest methods of meditation all surround achieving mindfulness. Achieving mindfulness is the most popular goal for meditators as it increases overall life satisfaction. Life satisfaction increases when you decrease stress, anxiety, and insomnia. Throughout this book, you will find tips and guides on how to combat psychological challenges. You will learn the simplest form of meditation to incorporating meditation in all your day to day activities. You will begin to understand how meditation will help you begin learning to love yourself and let go of negative thoughts. You will learn how to achieve a non-judgmental state of mind that will free your mind to accept everybody.

Related to meditation is something called *visualization*. Visualization is a type of inner transformation that leads to seeing actual results in reality. Visualization is also a form of creative thinking where people can shape their lives using a specific purpose within their minds. The best part about the image is that a person may have envisioned that it doesn't have to rely upon the outer world's external events. It can depend entirely on a person's imagination and the act of manifesting certain things. This idea will become relevant in the next section when we begin practicing meditation.

Meditation Techniques

In this ten-step guide, we will be using a mix of visualization and meditation to guide you into focusing on your goals. This guide is very similar to what we learned with visualization; researchers have found that visualizing and meditating on the process of a person achieving their goals will help them to do it in real life. Try these following steps of guided meditation to help put your goal into the future:

11. Start by thinking of an area of your life in your mind. Choose something where you

have been struggling with, or you would like to change.
12. Now start to imagine the best possible outcome you would like to live in concerning the area you've selected. Imagine these 6 to 12 months from now. What is the reality that you are looking to achieve? Try not to get caught up with any negativity or limitations; instead, just allow yourself to imagine and get carried away with your strongest goals.
13. Focus your mind on connecting with just one goal you would like to achieve over the next three months. Make sure your goal is a good one and is as meaningful as possible. If you choose a goal that is not meaningful or doesn't hold a lot of weight, the result won't feel special for you. Make sure to choose something significant enough to feel a high sense of accomplishment and motivation for your next goal once you achieve this goal. Be sure to run your goal through the SMART acronym to ensure that it is a goal that is set up for success.
14. Now that you are starting to feel connected with the goal that you've set, try to imagine what your life will be like once you achieve the goal. Visualize a picture or movie and try to view it as if you are looking at it through your pair of eyes. Factor in all the other sensory perceptions to try to imagine the most real and positive feelings. Where are you? Who is with you? What are the things happening around you?

15. Now, begin to step out of that picture or movie you've imagined and begin to imagine yourself floating up in the air where you are sitting now while taking that imagery with you. Take a deep breath and as you breathe out, use your breath to give life to the image and fill it with intention and positive energy. Repeat this five times.
16. In this step, it is time to imagine yourself floating out into the future while imagining yourself dropping the imagery you've created for your goal down into your real-life below you at the exact time and date you've set for yourself to reach this goal.
17. Pay attention to the things that need to happen between then and now and how it is beginning to re-evaluate itself to support you in achieving that goal. Visualize this process and all those events to make it feel as realistic as possible.
18. Once you feel like that step is complete, bring your awareness back to the present, and with your eyes still shut, start to think about what steps you will need to take in the next few days that will help you move closer to achieving your goal.
19. Take a few more deep breaths to ground yourself to the present before opening your eyes. Before you forget, write down a list of steps that you need to take to achieve your goal or begin to write down your experience in your journal, so you don't forget.
20. In this last step, you will focus on taking action and staying focused. Make sure that

you are doing something that brings you closer to achieving your goal daily.

Use this meditation and visualization technique once a week after you first complete the steps. Doing this once a week helps you continue to move forward towards your end goal and help you bring your vision into real life. Seeing is believing, so using your mind and meditation can create the best future that you have imagined for yourself.

What Is Mindful Eating?

There are many activities in your life that you may not even think that meditation can impact. In this section, we will discuss how incorporating meditation techniques into the act of eating will help you change your relationship with food and develop healthier rituals around eating. This technique is called *mindful eating*. Mindful eating is a technique that is done which incorporates mindfulness with eating. This technique helps people combat common food-related disorders, including emotional eating and binge eating that are so prevalent in our fast-paced lives.

Mindful eating is important because eating is one of the tasks that we perform numerous times every day of our lives. When we do a certain task repeatedly, our bodies will naturally try to automate that action to save us energy. However, when we eat mindlessly, we don't pay attention to the way food tastes, what we're eating, and how quickly we consume it. This automation causes people to mistreat their bodies without knowing. Fear not, as I will teach you how to begin using mindful eating to your benefit and provide you with some exercises to help you begin incorporating this into your daily life.

The Benefits Of Mindful Eating

Forgetting to eat mindfully is something that most of our population struggles with, and they don't even know it. This struggle happens because our lives function at such a fast pace that we don't put much thought into the details surrounding the act of eating.

We typically find ourselves eating at work, in front of our computer, eating dinner in front of the TV, or eating during the commute to work! This seemingly insignificant detail is one of the leading factors contributing to today's obesity and eating disorder problem. To combat this, we need to improve our relationship with eating and our eating rituals. This improvement comes down to an ability to eat mindfully.

Overall, practicing mindful eating will enhance your enjoyment of meals, prevent overeating, help with digestion, reduce anxiety about food-related matters, and better the relationship that you have with eating and food.

When and How to Use Mindful Eating

The goal of mindful eating is to shift your mind's focus from external thoughts to thoughts of exploration and enjoyment of the eating experience itself. We do this to develop a new mindset around food and a new relationship with food and the act of eating.

Here are a couple of points to come back to that will help you identify when you are eating mindlessly and switch to a mindful eating form.

1. You are consistently eating until the point of being full or even feeling physically il
2. You tend to nibble on snacks but don't taste them
3. You aren't don't notice what you eat, and you often find yourself eating meals in places that surround you with distractions
4. You are rushing through your meals
5. You have trouble remembering what you ate, or even the taste and smell of the last meal you've consumed

If you find yourself relating to any or all of the points that I just mentioned, you will surely benefit from mindful eating.

The Mindful Eating Technique

I will now share the technique of mindful eating with you. Next time you sit down for a meal, follow these tips to practice mindful eating and try to make it a daily habit.

12. Prioritize your mealtimes. Try to isolate a 15-minute block to take a seat and savour your food.

13. Be sure to get rid of any distractions present while you eat. You cannot enjoy the food you eat when you are not focused on it. Try asking yourself how often you eat sitting in front of the TV, in the car, or in front of the computer? Under those circumstances, eating is always mindless which can make you overeat, choose unhealthy foods for yourself, or neglecting to enjoy the food you are eating.
14. Try not to rush during meal times. Plan a time block in which you will eat, and make sure that you don't have any distractions around you. Even eating with a coworker or a friend may be a distraction due to conversation.
15. Always sit down to eat your meal. Try and avoid eating while standing up or walking as these create distractions.
16. Serve your meal on a plate or bowl. If possible, serve it on your favorite plate or bowl. Avoid eating food from the packet or take out containers as it makes eating feel less formal.
17. Ensure that you chew each bite thoroughly. Many people find themselves swallowing too soon and end up with digestion problems. Give your stomach an easier time digesting by breaking down the food properly before swallowing.
18. Make sure to only eat until you're 80% full. This level is a fine line. Don't eat until you are certain you are full, but eat until you feel satisfied. A lot of the time, the feeling of

fullness comes 10 minutes after you finish your meal. If you find yourself feeling full while you are still eating, you probably have overeaten.
19. Take your time to truly savor the taste of food. Use all five of your senses. Before eating, take a look at your meal of its look, smell, and overall appeal. Think about how each ingredient was cooked and seasoned and how you think the dish would taste because of it. During the meal, identify the taste of all the ingredients. What is the flavor? How does the flavor change if I eat different combinations of the ingredients? What does it smell like? What does the texture feel like on your tongue?
20. Think about how the meal is making you feel. Is it happy? Pleasurable? Guilty? Regretful? Stressed out? Disappointed? Pay attention to the thoughts that the food leads you to think. Do you think about specific memories? Fearful thoughts? Beliefs about anything? How does your body feel after the meal compared to before? Do you feel energetic after the meal, or does it make you tired? Is your stomach empty or full?
21. Try to make meals for yourself instead of buying them, when possible. The act of preparing food is proven to be psychologically beneficial and therapeutic. Make sure you are touching, tasting, and smelling the individual ingredients.
22. Make a note of the difference in good food. This difference tends to be food that is fresh,

seasonal, and minimally processed. Fresh and organic food tends to improve your overall mood and health. Food is our body's nourishment, and it provides the nutrition necessary for us to function optimally. Ingesting better quality food and ingredients is crucial to helping you feel better physically and psychologically.

Practicing meditation is your first step in being able to achieve mindful eating. Allowing yourself to be mindful in your day-to-day life will bring new joys and satisfactions that have always been there but have not been noticed in some time.

Chapter 5: Food-Related Changes to Begin Making

This chapter will provide you with a solid foundation of knowledge on which to build your new lifestyle. We will look at how intuitive eating can answer all of your struggles and help you find recovery.

Making Good Food-Related Choices

As we discussed earlier in this book, making good choices begins with self-exploration and a deep look into your core wounds. Once you have done this, you can begin to make positive decisions for your health and life, and over time these will become more and more habitual. We will spend this chapter looking at some of how you can begin to make good choices related to food and eating.

How to Begin Making Good Choices Using Intuitive Eating

One great way to make good choices when it comes to food is by using something called intuitive eating. Below, I will define intuitive eating for you and give you insight into how this can change your life.

What Is Intuitive Eating?

Intuitive eating is a new perspective from which to view how you feed your body. This eating style puts you in control. Instead of following a list of pre-

designed guidelines about when and what to eat. Intuitive eating encourages you to listen to your body and listen to the signals it sends you regarding;
- what to eat
- how much to eat
- when to eat.

Paying attention to these signals ensures that you are giving your body exactly what it needs when it needs it, instead of forcing it into a specific kind of diet.

Intuitive eating does not limit any specific foods and does not require you to exclusively stick to certain foods. Instead, it encourages you to learn as much as you can about what your body is telling you and follow its signals.

The two main components of the intuitive eating philosophy are eating when you are hungry and stopping eating when you are satiated. This concept may seem like a no-brainer, but we are very far from eating intuitively, as odd as it may seem in today's societies. With so many diet trends and numerous "rules" for how you should and should not eat, it can be difficult to put these ideas aside and let your body guide you exclusively.

The philosophy behind intuitive eating is that if you wait until you are too hungry before eating, you will be much more likely to overeat or binge eat. You should do this because, by this time, you be feeling ravenous instead of mildly hungry. If, instead, you choose to adhere to your hunger and eat when your body tells you that it needs sustenance, you will be much more likely to eat just the right amount. As a result, your body will be satisfied rather than completely stuffed, and instead of feeling shameful and angry that you have eaten, you can feel happy that you have provided your body with what it needed. This act requires you to listen to and respect what your body is telling you and then provide it with nutrients to keep working hard for you!

The Benefits of Intuitive Eating

One of the reasons that intuitive eating is such a successful and cherished form of eating is that it allows the body to lead the mind in the right direction when seeking out its needs. Below, we will look at the benefits of letting your body guide your eating choices.

- Allows the body to get what it needs

Did you know that your cravings could be giving you much more information than you give them credit for?

A craving is an intense longing for something (in this case food), that comes about intensely and feels urgent. In our case, that longing is for s a very specific type of food. When we have cravings for certain foods, it can mean more than what it seems.

While you may think that craving is an indication of hunger or a desire for the taste of a certain food, it may indicate that your body is low on certain vitamins or minerals. As a result, your body seeks out a certain food that it thinks will provide it with this vitamin or mineral. This requirement reaches your consciousness in the form of an intense craving. In this case, the body is trying to help itself by telling you what to eat. For this reason, understanding your cravings could help you give your body exactly what it is longing for.

For example, if you are craving juice or pop or other sugary drinks like this, consider that you might, in fact, be dehydrated and, therefore, thirsty. Sometimes we see drinks in our fridge, and since we are thirsty, we want them. Next time you are craving a sugary drink, try having a glass of water first, then wait a few minutes and see if you are still craving that Coca-Cola. You may not want it anymore once your thirst is quenched.

If you are craving meat, you may feel like you want some fried chicken or a hot dog. This craving could indicate a deficit of iron or protein. The best protein sources are chicken breast cooked in the oven, and iron is best received from spinach, oysters, or lentils. If you think you may not like these foods, there are many different ways to prepare them, and you can likely find a way you like.

- Prevents overeating

It can be hard to know how much to eat and when you have had enough to eat without letting yourself eat too much. Sometimes people will eat until the point that they begin to feel full. Often, we keep eating until we become stuffed, even to the point of making ourselves feel physically ill. Intuitive eating will help you avoid this, as this kind of eating encourages you to give your body what it needs to take great care of it. Stuffing your body until it is too full is not what your body is asking for, and once you become accustomed to listening to your body's needs, you will know when it is time to stop.

- Helps you break free from self-judgment

Intuitive eating will help you to finally make peace with your body and yourself as a whole. It does this by showing you that your body has needs and that there is no shame intending to these needs, as long as you do so in a healthy way.

You cannot fully embrace and practice intuitive eating if you have those nagging feelings of self-judgment each time you take a bite of food or decide that you will eat lunch when you are hungry. For this reason, to practice intuitive eating, you must understand that feeding your body is an act of compassion for yourself and that this does not need to come with self-judgment.

- It is inclusive, not exclusive.

One of the great things about this eating style is that it is not founded on restricting a person's intake of certain foods or allowing only a small variety of foods.

Diets like this are extremely hard to transition to and are hard to maintain for a long period. Intuitive eating is about including as many natural whole foods as you wish while also ensuring that you consume enough of your nutrients. With this style of eating, you can eat whatever you wish, whenever you wish. This part makes it much easier to stick with this type of diet and reduces the chances of falling off after a short period due to cravings or intense hunger. It does not restrict calories or reduce your intake greatly, making it easier to handle than a traditional diet for many people. It feels natural to eat in this way, which makes it effective.

How to Make Intuitive Eating Part of Your Life

One of the best ways to make this type of eating a part of your life is to practice it with intention. This intention is especially important when you are just beginning. Each time you feel a pang of hunger or a compulsion to eat, take a minute to examine your inner world. By doing this, you will get your mind and body accustomed to working together. Also, do the same after you eat. By doing these two things, you will ensure that you are eating when hungry and stopping when satisfied.

When you finish eating a meal, rank your fullness level on a scale of 1 to 10, 1 being extremely hungry and ten being extremely stuffed. This ranking will help you determine if you are successfully stopping when you are satisfied and not overeating.

It is also important that you learn how to deal with your emotions and feelings effectively without using food. Using the techniques you have learned in this book, you will address your inner demons, making space for you to listen to your body and its needs.

As you know by now, listening to your body, your emotions, and your mind is extremely important when it comes to practicing intuitive eating. As long as you remember this, you will be well on your way to becoming a lifelong intuitive eater.

What Kind of Foods Should You Choose?

Fish is a great way to get healthy fats into your diet. Certain fish are very low in carbohydrates but high in good fats, making them perfect for a healthy diet. They also contain minerals and vitamins that will be good for your health. Salmon is a great fish to eat, as it is versatile and delicious. Many fish also include essential fatty acids that we can only get through our diet. Other fish that are good for you include:
- Sardines
- Mackerel
- Herring
- Trout
- Albacore Tuna

Meat and Poultry make up a large part of most Americans' diets. Meats and Poultry that are fresh and not processed do not include any carbohydrates and contain high protein levels. Eating lean meats helps to maintain your strength and muscle mass and gives you energy for hours. Grass-fed meats, in particular, are rich in antioxidants.

Eggs are another amazing, protein-filled food. Eggs help your body feel satiated for longer and keep your blood sugar levels consistent, which is great for overall health. The whole egg is good for you, as the yolk is where the nutrients are. The cholesterol found within egg yolks also has been demonstrated to lower your risk of getting diseases like heart diseases, despite what most people think. Therefore, do not be afraid of the egg yolk!

Legumes are a great source of protein and fiber, and there are many different types to choose from. These include the following:
- All sorts of beans, including black beans, green beans, and kidney beans
- Peas
- Lentils of all colors
- Chickpeas
- Peas

Examples of fruits that you can eat include the following:
- Citrus fruits such as oranges, grapefruits, lemons, and limes
- Melons of a variety of sorts
- Apples
- Bananas
- Berries including strawberries, blueberries, blackberries, raspberries, and so on
- Grapes

Vegetables are a great source of energy and nutrients, and they include a wide range of naturally

occurring vivid colors, which should all be included in your diet.
- Carrots
- Broccoli and cauliflower
- Asparagus
- Kale
- All sorts of peppers, including hot peppers, bell peppers
- Tomatoes
- Root vegetables (that are a good source of healthy, complete carbohydrates) such as potatoes, sweet potatoes, all types of squash, and beets.

Seeds are another great source of nutrients, vitamins, and minerals, and they are very versatile. These include the following:
- Sesame seeds
- Pumpkin seeds
- Sunflower seeds
- Hemp, flax, and chia seeds are all especially good for your health

Nuts are a great way to get protein if you choose not to eat meat or vegan. They also are packed with nutrients. Some examples are below.
- Almonds
- Brazil Nuts
- Cashews
- Macadamia nuts
- Pistachios
- Pecans

Some healthy fats are essential components of any person's diet, as our bodies cannot make the beneficial compounds that they contain; thus, we rely solely on our diet to get them. These compounds are Omega-3 Fatty Acids, monounsaturated and polyunsaturated fats. Below are some healthy sources of these compounds:
- Avocados
- Healthy, plant-based oils including olive oil and canola oil
- Hemp, chia, and flax seeds
- Walnuts

When it comes to carbohydrates, these should be consumed in **whole grains**, as they are high in fiber, which will help prevent overeating. Whole grains also include essential minerals- those that we can only get from our diet, just like those essential compounds found in healthy fats. These essential minerals are selenium, magnesium, and copper. Sources of these whole grains include the following:
- Quinoa
- Rye, Barley, buckwheat
- Whole grain oats
- Brown rice
- Whole grain bread can be hard to find these days in the grocery store, as many brown loaves of bread disguise themselves as whole grain when, in fact, they are not. However, there are whole grain loaves of bread if you take the time to look at the ingredients list.

Electrolytes

When you first begin losing weight, having Electrolyte depletion is quite common. This depletion is because of water weight loss through fat, thus reducing electrolytes present in your body. Taking electrolyte supplements can help avoid a deficiency in common electrolytes, like magnesium, potassium, and sodium. This depletion is also why you should ensure you are getting enough dietary sodium, as this is an electrolyte that you need. Along with this, though, you will need to ensure you are drinking enough water to avoid dehydration.

Vitamin D

Vitamin D is found in some foods that have been fortified with it, but it can be found in only a few foods in a natural sense. These include cheese, fatty fish like salmon and tuna, as well as egg yolks. Another source is mushrooms that have been exposed to UV rays, so the organic ones are likely of this sort.

Vitamin D can be absorbed naturally through sun exposure, so if you live in a sunny place, make sure you get out for some walks or some timer with the sun on your skin. If you live in a colder or more gloomy place, consider purchasing a lamp that mimics the sun and provides you with vitamin D in your house. On a sunny day, even if it is cold, going outside and getting sun on your face will give you vitamin D.

Chapter 6: Weight Loss

Weight loss is never an easy task, and having the right mindset is crucial to your success, as we have seen throughout this book. Throughout this chapter, we will learn about weight loss and how best to set yourself up for success in this way!

Weight loss is something many people are chasing in the world today, but many of them are going about it in all of the wrong ways. Below, we will look at how you can achieve weight loss without using diets and how this relates to intuitive eating and exercise.

How to Achieve Weight Loss Without Using Diets

A combination of intuitive eating and exercise is the best way to achieve weight loss without using diets! As you have seen, intuitive eating is the best way to get in touch with your inner self, which this book is all about. Below, we will learn about the science of weight loss to better understand how it works within your body.

By taking control of your thoughts and beliefs, they don't have the opportunity to manifest into unhealthy behaviors such as overeating, turning to food for comfort, or any other unhealthy coping mechanisms that you have developed throughout your life. This concept is a through-line in this book, and it is something that I want you to remember for the rest of your life. You do not need diets to find a healthier you!

The Science of Weight Loss

If you are reading this book to lose weight, you will need to ensure that you understand the science of weight loss. The basic mathematical equation to represent weight loss is the following;

Calories in – (minus) Calories used for basic survival (for example, walking, eating, breathing) - (minus) Calories burned from exercise = (equals)

The number that results from this equation (in the equals position) will either be positive or negative.

- If the number is positive, this means that you ingested more calories than you burned. If the number is positive, you can envision it as having more energy than you could use. When this occurs, the extra energy is stored as fat in the body.
- If the number is negative, this means that you burned more calories than you ingested. If the number is negative, you used more energy than you had, which translates to weight loss. This effect happens because once the readily available energy in your body is all used up, the body's fat storage will begin to be used for additional energy, resulting in a loss of weight in the form of fat.
- If the number is zero, calories ingested and calories burned are equal. If the number is zero, this indicates "breaking even" in terms of your energy.

This equation explains how falling off the diet for one meal or two each day could lead to the maintenance of the same weight or even an increase in weight in some cases. This equation also shows us that weight gain or weight loss comes down to a simple mathematical equation that we must keep in mind. I am not sharing this to cause stress rather; to show you that you are in control of your weight loss journey.

How to Develop and Maintain a Healthy Diet Without Dieting

In diet culture, hunger is seen as an enemy. When it comes to intuitive eating, hunger is not an enemy but rather a source of information for you regarding what your body is asking for and what it needs. Instead of seeing hunger as an enemy, I want you to begin listening to your hunger. The philosophy behind this is that if you wait until you are too hungry before you eat, you will be much more likely to overeat because you will feel ravenous and want to eat everything in sight. If, instead, you choose to adhere to your hunger and eat when your body tells you that it needs sustenance, you will be much more likely to eat just the right amount, and you and your body will be satisfied rather than completely stuffed afterward. Instead of feeling shameful and angry that you are feeling hungry, feel happy that your body is telling you what it needs and that you can provide it with nutrients for it to keep working hard for you!

The above concept is how you can lose weight and begin to eat healthier without following a diet or giving in to any diet culture norms proven to be very harmful to people's mental health.

The diet industry may seem like it is in place to help you improve your life and become a better version of yourself, when in fact, it is banking on the fact that you never find success, as this will keep you coming back to spend more money and buy more books. When it comes to being healthy and taking good care of your body, intuitive eating cannot be thought of in the same way as a diet can, it should instead be seen as a philosophy that aims to help you return to the normal way that humans are meant to eat.

The diet industry is focused on making you feel like you are not perfect enough. Taking an approach focused on perfection leaves you feeling down on yourself and like a failure most of the time. Since this method leaves you feeling as though you are always short of perfection (instead of focusing on the positives), the progress you have made will always feel like it is still not enough, no matter how far you have come or how much progress you have made. Since you will never achieve perfection- as this is impossible for anyone, you will never feel satisfaction or celebrate your achievements. You will forever be chasing the "right diet" when, in fact, there is no right diet.

Intuitive eating, as discussed in the previous chapter, can be seen as the anti-diet mentality!

How to Shift Your Mind Toward Weight Loss

Intuitive eating is a good choice for anyone, especially for those who prefer more flexibility when it comes to their eating time and those who do not want to restrict their eating at all. Humans should not be putting themselves through boot camp every time they feel hungry, and this method does not adhere to that type of mindset.

One of the reasons that intuitive eating is such a successful and cherished form of eating is that it allows the body to lead the mind in the right direction when seeking out its needs. For example, did you know that your cravings could be giving you much more information than you give them credit for? Below we will look at what your cravings could mean and why this means that you should let your body guide your eating choices.

By beginning to view your life in this way, you will not fight against your body and mind, but instead, learn to work along with them. This change will help you to achieve a sense of harmony.

Chapter 7: Learning to Love Exercise

Exercise is great for your body, your mind, and your overall health. Adding an exercise regime into your life is as important, if not more, than any other measures you take to maintain your health. For this reason, we will spend an entire chapter learning about how to love exercise and make it a regular part of your life! This chapter will learn about the importance of making peace with your body and how you can begin to do this.

The Benefits of Exercise for Your Mental Health

Exercise has been proven to help with various things in life, such as stress, impotence, and mental health. Exercise will help you in your journey to recovery because of how it affects the different systems of your body. As you know, all of our body systems work together to form the person that we are. If one of them isn't functioning quite as well as it should be, all of the other systems feel the negative effects.

Exercise works on all of your body systems simultaneously. If one of them isn't firing on all cylinders, exercise will help that system feel better because the movement is nothing but healthy for the mind and body.

Exercising will help you take your mind off those nagging cravings and give you a clearer mind overall with which you can look deep inside at those cravings and the emotional issues that are causing them. Exercise will help in all aspects of your life and will help you to continue reaching for recovery.

In addition to this, exercise has positive chemical effects on our minds. When we exercise, our brain releases chemicals that tell us that we enjoy the exercise's effects. This feeling is known as "runner's high," and it is that thrill you feel after you run a long-distance or complete a workout. When you are feeling down and exercise, your mood will lift because of this runner's high. For this reason, it is not so important what kind of physical exercise you do, but rather the fact that you engage in it regularly to help you feel motivated and to keep your mood positive. This runner's high can be compared to those rewarded feelings that the highly sugary foods give us, but with runner's high, the feeling of joy and accomplishment last way longer than the rewarded happy feelings we get from eating food. Industrial food makes our brains feel happy, but our body feels heavy and sluggish. As I mentioned, exercise makes all of our body parts feel great simultaneously, which is why the effects of runner's high are so long-lasting.

How to Begin Using Exercise to Your Benefit

Whether you are a seasoned exerciser or someone who has never exercised before, there is an exercise routine out there for you. Do not be discouraged by your experience level when it comes to exercise, as everyone can benefit from it, and everyone must start somewhere. Do not be discouraged by your experience level when it comes to exercise, as everyone can benefit from it, and everyone must start somewhere. This section will give you several ideas for exercise, no matter the experience level you bring with you, by teaching you about something called *intuitive movement.*

What Is Intuitive Movement?

Intuitive movement is the practice of moving according to the needs and wishes of your body. It can be thought of similarly to intuitive eating, except with the movement of your body instead.

Many people begin following some type of exercise plan to get in shape or to lose weight. This method does not often lead to success, as people often have to try to force themselves to perform exercise that doesn't feel good for their body, which has not been personalized for them, and which they find no enjoyment in. This determination often lasts for a week or two, after which the person becomes fed up and decides that having to push themselves to perform the exercise plan is not worth the potential benefits.

On the other hand, intuitive movement involves a deeper motivation and an enjoyment factor not often present in other kinds of exercise regimes. If you enjoy the movement, you are much more likely to want to perform it, and you will not even need to force your body to do it, as you will genuinely want to take part in it.

There are so many forms of movement available for our bodies, regardless of our skills or experience levels. Below, I will share several types of exercise and their benefits so that you can choose the type of movement that suits you best.

Cardiovascular Exercise Versus Resistance Training

Cardiovascular exercise and resistance training are two different types of exercise that people can benefit from. Cardiovascular exercise is the type of exercise that involves an elevated heart rate due to activities such as running, riding a bicycle, or swimming. This type of exercise is often referred to as "cardio." This type of exercise is usually done for an extended period at a steady state.

Resistance training is a type of exercise that involves using weights to build up your muscles by doing things like squats, push-ups, bicep curls, and so on. This exercise is the type of exercise you would often do if you go to a gym to exercise. Contrary to popular belief, this type of exercise will not make you bulky and muscular, especially if you are a woman. Instead, it will give you more tone and a leaner body.

When we engage in cardiovascular exercise, our heart rate increases; what this does is carry more oxygen to our muscles so that they can keep exercising. It also carries more oxygen to our brain. More oxygen and blood flow to the brain means that your brain will work more efficiently, more sharply, and with more clarity, after you finish exercising. More blood flow to the brain also means that it will be generally healthier. Exercising often and for a continuous period helps keep the brain structures themselves healthy and in working order. Exercise helps with memory, decision making, and learning. Exercise is the most effective antidepressant. Many pills are prescribed to treat and beat depression, but the most effective and most natural way to continually boost your mood and keep it up is through exercise. The effects that exercise has on the brain are far-reaching and numerous.

When we exercise, we become stronger, faster, and more agile. These benefits not only help us to exercise better but it helps us in our everyday lives. Moving through life with more ease than before is a great feeling that can only be achieved through exercise. Our bodies are built to move, and they love it when we do move! Our bodies are built to continually become stronger with the more we do, and this is what inevitably happens as soon as we begin exercising regularly.

You can begin to see aesthetic changes as well. You can see your muscles growing, your body toning, and your fast disappearing. These changes on the inside and outside make us feel great about the body we live in and the progress we are making mentally.

Taking the time to exercise and stick with an exercise regime shows our body that we are willing to do the hard work that exercising takes, and it also shows our mind the same thing.

The Benefits of Other Kinds of Exercise

Numerous other exercises do not fit into one of the two categories as described above. These include exercises such as yoga, Pilates, high-intensity interval training, group training classes, and so on. While these are not considered traditional exercise methods, they are no less valid than resistance training or cardiovascular exercise. Many people who are not too enthused about exercise wish to pursue methods that incorporate more social aspects or slower movements. If this is what you prefer, this is just as valid as going for a run!

There are even more ways to be active such as pursuing activities like gardening, dancing, hiking, kayaking, etc. Any activity that gets your heart rate raised and brings you a sense of joy and accomplishment can be used as an exercise combined with a diet change to bring you weight loss results!

If you normally don't do much exercise or walk around often, begin by taking the stairs sometimes. Begin by deciding to walk some places, like down the street or around the block. Beginning with this type of movement will get your body used to moving again and will get your muscles and joints moving smoothly.

If you occasionally walk, like to a bus stop or the store on your lunch break, you can begin with a little bit more exercise than someone who is sedentary. Since your muscles and joints are likely somewhat used to being in a standing position, you can begin to jog a little bit. You can jog after dinner around the block a few times or jog to the store and walk back every few days. You could also take a yoga class if you wish or do some video-guided yoga at home.

If you have a moderate level of walking in your life and occasionally speed up to a jog, you can begin to move your body around in new and different ways. Try doing sit-ups and push-ups at home before or after your run or run to the park and use the playground equipment to do some chin-ups, some two-foot jumps onto a step, or run up and down the steps a few times. Doing this will keep your heart rate up and teach your body new ways of moving while allowing your upper body muscles to get a bit of attention as well.

If you run frequently and have some bodyweight exercise sessions now and again, try visiting a gym and doing some more weight exercises. You can try squatting, pressing some things overhead, and maybe some bicep curls. Doing this will challenge your muscles in ways that your body weight cannot and take you to a new level of fitness and mood-boosting.

If you are an experienced runner, you are likely quite familiar with the feeling of runner's high. You are likely quite familiar with how exercise can change your mood and take you from feeling hopeless to hopeful. If you want to try some new forms of exercise, try creating a routine in the gym lifting weights. Doing this will take your running to new heights and will give you a new type of exercise experience to break up the running days.

Suppose you are experienced when it comes to exercise, good for you! Continue to challenge yourself in new ways and teach your body new ways of moving. Exercise does nothing but good things, so keep up your routine.

Since exercising helps women regain some of the muscle mass lost due to age, it can be greatly beneficial for women to exercise into their older years. It is important to be aware of how to do this safely, though. It can be safer to stick to low-impact exercises, so exercises that avoid jumping or any sort of quick, jarring movements. Instead, spending some time on an exercise bike (or a real bike) or elliptical machine can be good as they reduce impact and are therefore better for a woman's joints. Things like running involve more impact, so if you have joint pain, it is best to avoid this type of exercise. Further, lifting some small weights or walking with weights in your hands can help you build back some muscle. Building muscle will lead to an increase in your resting rate of metabolism (the number of calories your body burns when it is just sitting, at rest to execute living functions such as breathing or sitting). The increase will greatly improve your overall health in muscle, improve your joint health, and the lowered risk of diseases such as heart disease (which is reduced by doing aerobic exercise). Staying active in your 50's is a great decision, and every capable woman should add exercise into their lives, regardless of the diet they follow.

How Exercise Can Change Your Relationship With Your Body

Exercise meets you where you are, and your brain will gladly take any new form of movement as a mood booster. When you enjoy the exercises that you are taking part in, you are much more likely to choose to engage in them more often and much less likely to find excuses to avoid them. By enjoying what you are doing, it will feel like a reward and not like a punishment. For this reason, be sure to choose a form of exercise (or multiple forms) that you enjoy.

Exercising while on this process to recovery will help you feel strong both physically and mentally when your journey may be getting tough. Exercising will show you what your body can do, and how strong it is, making you feel stronger mentally.

The Importance of Sleep

You may have heard before that sleep is essential to a person's success in every aspect of their life, but you may not know why this is. A person's sleep cycle has been proven to have strong effects on their mood and their willpower. When a person does not get enough sleep, their symptoms of depression, or their negative mood, in general, have been shown to worsen.

Sleep deprivation causes other negative symptoms like sadness, fatigue, moodiness, and irritability. When you are trying to pursue a lifestyle change, including incorporating more exercise and changing your diet, you need to maintain a positive mood to remain motivated and track to accomplish your goals.

Since the theory behind willpower is that it requires energy from the brain to be maintained, and the brain restores its energy from a restful sleep, it's safe to assume that sleep is directly connected to the level of willpower that a person can exercise. When a person doesn't get enough sleep, their brain spends most of its energy focused on keeping the body's basic functions up and running (such as walking, breathing, and moving. These energy demands do not leave much energy for a person to spend on exerting their willpower, practicing self-discipline, or simply remembering their goals.

Getting a proper and healthy amount of sleep is vital for accomplishing anything, especially if those things are challenging. When a person doesn't get enough sleep, it affects their ability to focus, judgment, mood, overall health, and diet.

When people suffer chronic sleep deprivation such as insomnia, things go from bad to worse. Many research studies have found evidence that people who don't get the proper amount of sleep regularly have a greater risk of catching specific diseases. Lack of sleep also has a significant and negative impact on a person's immune system. This impact can cause a person to frequently catch colds or flu cases that cause them not to go to school, work, or get anything effective done.

Not many people can function well with less than seven hours of sleep per night. A healthy adult should be aiming for 7 – 9 hours of sleep every night. For an adult, it is important to get at least six hours of sleep every night. A healthy amount of sleep should range between eight to ten hours every night, but the minimum requirement is 6 hours. To ensure you are getting this much sleep, avoid eating or drinking anything that contains caffeine for at least 5 hours before bedtime so that it doesn't affect your natural sleep cycle. Make a note to also stay away from ingesting too many toxins during the day such as cigarettes, alcohol, drugs, or prescription medicine if it can be avoided, as these can lead to a reduction in sleep quality.

The benefits of getting enough sleep are extraordinary. Aside from the fact that it can help you stay focused and be more disciplined, it also helps with the following;

- curbing inflammation and pain
- lowering stress
- improving your memory
- jumpstarting your creativity

- sharpening your attention
- improving your grades
- limiting your chances of accidents
- helping you avoid negative feelings that can lead to depression or anxiety.

Chapter 8: Using Affirmations

This chapter will learn about a great strategy that will prove useful to you in helping you reach your weight loss goals. This tool can help you because of the positive mental state that it can put you in, and because of the increase in self-esteem it can bring you. This tool is something called an *Affirmation*.

What Are Affirmations?

Affirmations are, by definition, spoken or written phrases, which state something to be true. More specifically, affirmations are the valuable and uplifting assurances that we tell ourselves. They are words or phrases that we use to state something about ourselves or our lives to be true.

Declarations are similar to affirmations in that they are the act of declaring something. The difference between affirmations and declarations is that declarations can be an opinion or a belief rather than a fact. The word declaration can be used as a noun or as a verb, as in *to make a declaration*, which is when you share your declaration with others in the form of writing or speaking.

We will look at some examples of affirmations and declarations below, and I will teach you how to make some for yourself to use in your own life. Please note that from here forward, we can use the terms affirmation and declaration interchangeably.

How Affirmations Will Benefit You

The technique of implementing change that lasts is to change the way someone perceives themselves. So how does affirmation play a role here? Affirmations are very effective when used out loud so that you can hear the positive reminders being said in your voice. Humans naturally believe the things that they tell themselves. For example, if someone dislikes some aspect of their physical appearance, they will believe that they are unattractive. The next time you are in front of a mirror, practice using affirmations by saying something you like about yourself. By repeating this every time, you are in front of a mirror will eventually lead you to believe these positive things, and you will begin to focus on the positive rather than what you don't like about yourself.

How to Use Affirmations

If someone is trying to improve their self-esteem or their negative mind state, the affirmations they use should be focused solely on positive things.

Suppose a person wishes to use affirmations to achieve specific goals. In that case, it is beneficial for them to use affirmations that remind them of their positive personal values and their potential.

Try repeating your affirmations aloud to yourself, or even writing them down (or better yet, a combination of both) frequently. Doing this will help you build a positive self-narrative that will lead to an increase in your level of self-esteem over time and, thus, a greater likelihood of achieving your goals.

We will look at the steps you will need to take to create your own affirmations below, and once you have created them for yourself, you will be ready to begin using them right away. Once you have completed your positive affirmations, schedule a block of time every day or a couple of times per week to take a look back at them and update them. The more you read them and drill them into your memory, the more positive thoughts will naturally come to you. You can also document any changes you feel in yourself as you do this exercise.

How to Come up With Affirmations of Your Own

8. **Structure your affirmation** To begin, you want to structure your affirmation so that it begins with something called an *"I statement."* This point means that you want to start your sentence with *"I am..."*

9. **Focus on creating affirmations that have a positive outcome**.
Try to refrain from using avoidant words such as "not" in your statements. Make them as positive as you can, as your brain feels positive when it hears positive words like "can!"

10. **Keep your affirmations as concise as you can.**

Ensure they are concise, so they guide you to the point and serve as quick reminders of positivity.

11. **Design your affirmations to be as specific as possible**.

This point is especially important if it guides you to your goal, as you want to ensure that you are keeping yourself focused on the goal so that you are continuously reminding yourself of it.

12. **Try to write your affirmations in the present tense**.

Focus on using a word that ends with "ing" this will help you ensure that you are using the word's present tense.

13. **Use descriptive words**

Using descriptive words will give your affirmation more impact and will make it more detailed.

14. **Make your affirmations personal to you and your situation**.

Ensure that your affirmations relate to your specific goals or whatever you are dealing with at the moment; this will increase their impact when you use them and help you remember why you are using them.

Chapter 9: Hypnosis Techniques for Weight Loss

In this chapter, we will discuss the topic of hypnosis and how it can benefit you in this weight loss journey that you are embarking on.

What Is Hypnosis?

Hypnosis is the practice of reaching an altered state of consciousness where a person is said to lose control of their actions and is very susceptible to the power of suggestion or to being given direction. This technique is done to achieve new behaviors or thoughts that were previously difficult to grasp or understand. This method is also done to break tough habits or addictions, such as an addiction to smoking cigarettes.

This practice works because this altered state of consciousness allows a person to become more open-minded and receptive to suggestions. Without hypnosis, a person may be resistant to accepting new thoughts or concepts, and they may be closed off to new ideas or trying new behaviors. If these are introduced in a hypnosis state, the person will be much more open to them, and when they return to a normal state of consciousness, they will be left with these imprinted ideas, beliefs, or behaviors. This method works because it taps into the subconscious mind, where the conscious mind cannot step in and inhibit the absorption of concepts or ideas that it decides it does not want. By programming these new ideas and thoughts into the subconscious mind, your body can act according to thoughts you are unaware of, and this is how new beliefs or behaviors can come about before you can stop them.

The altered state of consciousness achieved by undergoing hypnosis is similar to the state that is achieved in the moments before a person falls asleep. In these moments, a person is said to be the most creative, relaxed, and open-minded.

The Benefits Of Hypnosis

Hypnosis has proven beneficial for removing negative beliefs or thought patterns, including limiting beliefs and replacing them with new positive or beneficial beliefs. This practice is especially effective for those stubborn and deep-seated beliefs and habits that you have been trying to kick but have been unable to. Since you now understand that deep emotional struggles often cause weight gain and obesity, you can see how hypnosis can help a person overcome those struggles and lose weight for good.

In addition to the above benefits, hypnosis has been shown to reduce pain, reduce anxiety, and bring about a sense of calm to a person. It can also improve your sleep quality and improve Irritable Bowel Syndrome (IBS) symptoms, which affects a large portion of the population.

For our specific purposes, hypnosis is beneficial for several reasons. It allows a person to become receptive to the power of suggestion; it can help a person cast off their negative self-image and see themselves positively.

Further, it can help break the cycle of emotional eating by dealing with the root causes of this type of eating and can teach a person to turn to different methods of dealing with their feelings and emotions other than turning to food. This conscious choice can break the cycle of emotional eating; as I said in the previous chapter, the most effective way to deal with this is to examine the root causes and address those first. As this is very difficult to do for many people, especially if the root causes are painful to revisit, hypnosis can effectively access those deep feelings and fears to confront and deal with them. Hypnosis does this by removing the mental blocks that the conscious mind puts up to protect us from our negative feelings and fears.

There are three ways that you can change your emotional state whenever you wish to. These ways include changing yourself on a physical level, on a mental level, and finally, using verbal techniques. We will look at each of these three ways in more detail below, including how hypnosis can benefit you in each of these three ways.

   4. Physical

Hypnosis works at the physical level by helping you relax your body using deep breathing and a lowered cognition level.

   5. Mental

Hypnosis works to change your emotional state as it allows you to change your thought patterns, which changes your emotional state

6. Verbal

To change your emotional state using verbal techniques, you must employ methods such as the following
- Changing the words you use from negative to positive ones
- Listening to guided meditations (hypnosis) as a way to learn to employ new vocabulary

The Different Levels Of Consciousness

Hypnosis allows a person to reach different levels of consciousness that they otherwise may not be able to. You may be wondering what different levels of consciousness are possible with the human mind.

The Conscious Mind

The conscious mind includes everything that you are aware of. This state includes your thoughts, your short-term memories, and anything that is currently occupying your mind.

The Subconscious Mind

On the other hand, the subconscious mind is the part of your consciousness without your knowledge. This level includes things like memories, which are in your mind which you are not currently aware of, but which can be brought into your conscious mind any time you wish to access them.

The 5 Levels Of Consciousness

When it comes to hypnosis, there are considered to be five levels of consciousness. These different states of consciousness represent different levels of use of the conscious and the subconscious mind.

6. Gamma

The Gamma level of consciousness is that which is entered when brain activity is very high. This state includes times of fear, panic, and anxiety when thoughts in the conscious mind are running quickly from one to the next.

7. Beta

The Beta level of consciousness is the regular state of consciousness that you are in most of the time throughout your life. This stage includes a regular level of awareness of what you are doing and thinking and a regular brain activity level.

8. Alpha

Alpha level of consciousness can be said to be a *Daydream*-like state of mind. This level can be the early stages of hypnosis or when you are meditating. This level begins to include the subconscious mind.

9. Theta

This level is when the subconscious mind begins to take over. There is little conscious thought involved at this level, and you are in touch with the subconscious. This level is usually found during sleep and deeper states of meditation and hypnosis.

   10. Delta

The fifth and final level of consciousness is the Delta level. This level is the deepest, and it does not involve any conscious mind, and it involves a state of deep sleep or a deep trance. This state can be achieved during the deepest sleep levels or by people skilled and experienced with meditation and hypnosis.

How Can Hypnosis Help With Weight Loss?

Hypnosis effectively changes a person's body because it opens the mind to accepting and practicing new behaviors. By changing behaviors, a person can change their body. These behaviors include eating habits and exercise habits. Further, hypnosis can lead to release from negative thought patterns and negative body image. In turn, this practice can also lead to a reduction in the likelihood of emotional eating, as the mind and body will not be seeking comfort and feelings of reward like they were when the person's mind was wrought with negativity.

One of the first beliefs that we want to change through hypnosis is the negative beliefs that you have about your weight.

We want to address and change through hypnosis because of the negative beliefs you hold about weight loss and dieting and the negative beliefs you have about exercise.

We want to replace these negative beliefs with new positive and empowering ones so that you can begin to change your life as a whole.

Hypnosis For Cravings

Below we will look at how you can begin to change the negative thought processes that occur in your mind and how you can begin to reshape them to develop a new perspective of weight loss and diet using hypnosis.

By taking stock of your unhelpful thinking styles and your core wounds, you will begin to notice them as they come up in your mind throughout the day. By being able to do this, you can begin to turn them around by consciously combatting them and reminding yourself of your positive thinking styles. This practice will help you remain on track to achieving your goals and making this new lifestyle a habit. By doing this during the day, you are training your mind to reach for positive thoughts instead of negative ones over time. Eventually, those positive thoughts will happen more often than the unhelpful ones. This type is a form of self-hypnosis, as you are changing your beliefs and thoughts, which is one of the main goals of hypnosis.

Suppose you can get yourself into a daydream-like state several times during the day and, from there, shift your thinking toward positivity and goal-oriented thoughts. In that case, you can begin to allow your subconscious to feed you those positive thoughts throughout the day, which will help with your motivation and your daily pursuit of your weight loss and diet goals. By catching and changing your thoughts before they spiral out of control, you will be in control of your emotions and behavior as well.

By intervening in your natural thought progression when it comes to weight loss, you can change your thoughts regarding weight-loss into more positive and goal-oriented thoughts. For example, instead of thinking, "I will fail at weight loss because I always have in the past," You can instead jump in and change this automatic negative thought to something more positive. For example, "This time, I will succeed since I have set myself up for success by goal setting and reading this book." During hypnosis, you can change your negative fail-focused thoughts to more positive ones, which will lead these positive thoughts to come to the surface more readily in your daily life after that. Doing this will, in turn, inform your behavior and lead you to success.

Doing this can help you deal with nagging cravings because you can consciously choose to avoid them and instead make a healthier choice for yourself.

Self-Hypnosis

Self-Hypnosis, in contrast to other types of hypnotherapy, is done alone rather than with a therapist or a "hypnotizer" present. Self-hypnosis is done by getting yourself into a state of deep relaxation, to the point of allowing the subconscious mind to come to the surface and encouraging the conscious mind to take a back seat. When you get into a self-hypnosis state, you can then begin to introduce the suggestion portion of hypnosis- either in the form of suggesting new thoughts and behaviors to yourself or by listening to an audio guide for this exact purpose. These audioguides can be found online in a variety of places, one of which is YouTube. With self-hypnosis, you can use any form of hypnosis that you wish (any of those described above), according to the motivations for using hypnosis in the first place.

If you are just getting started with self-hypnosis, the best way to initiate this is by practicing mindfulness. We discussed mindfulness briefly in this book thus far, but here I will show you an example of how you can get into a state of mindfulness to begin self-hypnosis if you are not experienced with it.

Mindfulness and meditation go hand in hand. Meditation increases mindfulness while mindfulness improves and deepens meditation. Meditation is a practice, while mindfulness is a state of being.

To get into a state of mindfulness involves getting quiet and observing, without judgment, everything that occurs within your body. You must let your thoughts drift by, noticing but not judging them. Notice all of your body's physical feelings; is there any tension that you notice? Notice how breathing feels on a physical level. Feel any sensations that you are experiencing. Notice also your emotions and feelings. By doing this repeatedly, you will be able to eventually focus on your body with less and less distracting thoughts. When your thoughts start to distract you, bring your attention back to your body, and breathing. Being able to reach a state like this allows you to reconnect with your body from the inside. Approaching your body with a non-judgment mindset will also make it easier for you to change your beliefs about your body or introduce new thoughts and behaviors. Instead of letting your mind spiral with anxious *what-if* thoughts, you will not let them escalate. They will not escalate to the level they normally would because instead of judging yourself and your body and worrying about what is wrong with you, you will approach it as is and without trying to force anything.

By focusing on the body and letting your thoughts enter your consciousness one by one, you can untangle them, resulting in a reduction in stress level. The state of meditation also brings about a state of relaxation and calm. Often, we are running around with a mind full of running thoughts, one after the other. When we take time to sit in silence, breathe, and sort through everything we are thinking and feeling through a non-judgmental lens, it leads to a state of inner peace. This inner peace state makes it much easier for your body to let in and embrace the good feelings and allows your mind to be more open and receptive to them.

By trying this exercise several times, it will begin to come easier over time, and you will then be able to get into a state of self-hypnosis much quicker. Once you have reached this level, you can then practice any sort of hypnosis in the form of self-hypnotism.

Other Techniques

When it comes to hypnosis, there are a variety of different types that you can engage in. In this section, I will outline them to get a better idea of how they can be employed in your life to help you in your journey of self-discovery and weight loss.

- Cognitive Hypnotherapy

The first type of hypnotherapy that we will discuss is called *cognitive hypnotherapy*. The term *hypnotherapy* relates to hypnosis therapy, and these two terms (hypnotherapy and hypnosis) can be used interchangeably.

Cognitive hypnotherapy is a type of hypnosis that is focused on a person's beliefs. It aims to change these beliefs to free a person from their limiting beliefs. It encourages people to look at their lives and beliefs from a new perspective and re-evaluate them. This type of hypnosis is similar in many ways to traditional Cognitive Behavioral Therapy (CBT), a type of talk therapy used to treat people with a variety of mental health disorders that includes depression, anxiety, as well as PTSD (Post-Traumatic Stress Disorder). CBT's fundamentals are based on three components; cognition (thought), emotion, and behavior. All three components interact with each other in the human mind, which leads to the theory that our thoughts determine our feelings and emotions, which then determines our behavior. Again, this is further evidence of the mind-body connection at work. Cognitive Behavioral Therapy works by emphasizing the relationship between your thoughts, feelings, and behaviors. When you begin to change any of these three components, you begin to initiate change in the other two components. CBT aims to increase your life's overall quality by helping you examine it from a new perspective. In this way, cognitive hypnotherapy can be beneficial for our purposes here, as it aims to change behaviors through changing thoughts or addressing emotions.

- Behavioral Hypnotherapy

This type of hypnotherapy is one of the classic forms, as it is one of the first practiced hypnotherapies. This type of hypnotherapy is a great place to begin if a person has no hypnotherapy experience. It is less intrusive and mentally demanding than some other forms of hypnotherapy. As you can guess, this type is done to change people's behaviors by shifting the current behaviors to more positive ones. The therapist will get the patient into a state of hypnosis. Then they will begin to suggest and talk through alternative behaviors to introduce them into the person's subconscious mind, therefore solidifying them for the person.

- Regression Hypnotherapy

Regression hypnotherapy is one of the more demanding and intrusive types of hypnotherapy. It involves looking back into a person's memories in their subconscious mind to tackle the root causes of whatever problems or struggles the person is having. This kind of therapy relates to what we discussed in the first chapter of this book, where we looked at possible underlying causes of a negative internal environment.

By taking part in regression hypnotherapy, a person can revisit their past or childhood to determine what types of trauma or events led them to develop the problems they are looking to overcome.

This type of hypnotherapy is not done until a person is comfortable with the practice of hypnosis, and it comes with some risks, as it could lead a person to be re-traumatized. This practice should only be done with a therapist whom you trust and only after experiencing other hypnosis forms.

Visualization As A Form Of Self-Hypnosis

In this section, we will look at visualization and how this can come together with hypnosis to influence the mind, and therefore the body (thanks to the mind-body connection) to make lasting changes for the better.

What Is Visualization?

Most people have tried to visualize their goals at least a couple of times in their lives. They probably spend a lot of time visualizing a desired future event. For the general public, visualization is a process where they picture their future within their mind. However, visualization can be used for much more than just that. It is a type of inner transformation that leads to seeing actual results in reality. Visualization is also a form of creative thinking where people can shape their lives using a specific purpose within their minds. The best part about the image is that a person may have envisioned that it doesn't have to rely upon the outer world's external events. It can depend entirely on a person's imagination.

The Benefits Of Visualization

Here is something that not many people know: Visualizing an action or a skill before actually performing it is nearly as effective as physically doing it. Scientific studies found evidence of people's thoughts creating the exact same patterns of activity in their mind as it does with the physical movements of the action. When somebody is mentally rehearsing or practicing something in their mind using the visualization process, it impacts the many cognitive processes within a person's brain, including planning, motor control, memory, and attention perception. In layman's terms, the way a person's brain is stimulated when they visualize an action is the same as when they are performing it physically. Therefore, scientists can safely assume that the act of visualization provides just as much value as physically performing a task.

Many athletes in certain sports use the act of visualization to help themselves train before a competition. For example, in Olympic cycling, the cyclist will prepare for a competition by closing their eyes and visualizing the racetrack in their mind. They move their bodies while visualizing how they will travel through the racetrack to train their muscle memory and reflexes even further. This way, when they do begin to compete on the racetrack, they have already visualized themselves cycling through it using the strategies that they have been taught and visualized in their minds. This technique is a technique and training skill that many professional coaches teach their athletes to do.

When a person is visualizing, their conscious mind is aware that what they're visualizing is not real but is just a result of imagination. Consequently, a person's subconscious cannot differentiate the difference between what a person is thinking and what they are doing. In other words, a person's inner mind isn't able to distinguish the difference between real life, a photo, memories, or an imagined future. Rather, the mind is under the impression that everything a person sees is real. This fact is proven by numerous brain scans that scientists have conducted over the years. They discovered that there are no brain activity differences when someone observes something in the real world compared to when a person is visualizing.

All of this evidence is extremely important because it points to the theory that visualization can help people learn new skills and reprogram and rewire their brains without performing physical actions. For example, suppose somebody is looking to increase their self-esteem. In that case, they can use visualization by imagining themselves doing those actions before actually doing it in the real world.

How To Use Visualization

Below, I will outline several different examples of visualization practice that you can try in various scenarios. These visualization exercises can help you create an action plan to help you achieve your goals or begin putting a plan into action before taking physical action to achieve goals you have set out for yourself already.

Visualization for Creating a Plan of Action

It is normal to become stressed out or feel overwhelmed when trying to achieve new goals. For this reason, creating a plan of action using visualization can help you relax and motivate you to take action. This technique is most effective if you use it before you go to bed to start planning the next day. You can also use this technique anytime during the day, when you have 10 minutes of free time.

Below are three simple steps on how to do this:

4. Calm yourself down and make sure you are feeling relaxed. Sit down as it will help you get some rest from whatever you were doing before.
5. Close your eyes and start to visualize which things specifically that you want to accomplish for tomorrow. Now, visualize those actions that you'd like to do in as much detail as you can and then ask yourself these questions below:

    h) How would I like to feel?
    i) How may I act around others?
    j) Which specific actions do I want to take?
    k) What do I want?
    l) Which challenges may I face?
    m) How can I deal with these challenges?
    n) What results do I want to come from this?

6. The reality here is that people cannot predict all the things that might happen to them. When events happen unexpectedly, they can often ruin any plans that have been put in place. However, good planning isn't about planning around all possible obstacles, but it is more about adapting to the obstacles that life gives you. When you keep this in mind, you must affirm with yourself at the end of

your session with "this or something better will come my way." By giving yourself affirmation, you are keeping your mind open to endless possibilities. This practice will result in more ready and okay with making adjustments when unexpected things happen to you.

This process is not a foolproof plan. However, this visualization will help you envision possible situations that might happen. These scenarios will help you choose more ideal options for yourself as you continue to work towards your goals.

Visualization for Achieving Goals That You Have Set Out for Yourself

This visualization technique is the most important one when it comes to strengthening self-discipline. Using the visualization technique for setting goals brings a lot of value, but this technique does come with one major drawback. The most popular form of visualization is goal setting. Most people have used visualization pertaining to their goals at one time or another. However, this technique may not have worked for them due to one critical flaw. This flaw is that when people visualize their goals, they only focus on visualizing their end goal and nothing in between. They see within their mind's a big and flashy awesome goal that's going to be rainbows and butterflies. Yes, they are experiencing this using all of their senses, but they simply open their eyes after the visualization, feeling very inspired. However, this type of motivation is extremely short-lived because the next time this person faces an obstacle, it immediately deflates their motivation.

When this happens, people feel the imagine the same goal all over again to create extra motivation. Though, because nothing happens after visualizing again, their motivation does not grow either. In fact, every time a person hits an obstacle and tries the process of visualization again, their motivation becomes weaker every time, and they start to lose more and more energy.

The mistake that these people are making is that they are not properly visualizing their goals. They only see the destination, but they don't understand that achieving a goal takes much more than just that. Achieving a goal is part of a journey that is full of emotional highs and lows, wins and losses, and journey of ups and downs. Due to this, these are the things that a person would also need to include in their visualization.

When a person visualizes their end goal, it is very effective in creating that desire and hunger. However, the proper way to use visualization is to spend 10 percent of your time visualizing the end goal and spending the rest of the visualization time thinking about HOW you will achieve your goals and overcome challenges. In some ways, it's similar to the form of visualization planning that we just discussed.

A person's end goal helps keep inspiration running in the long term, but it is the journey that helps a person stay motivated in the short term. To maximize the time spent on achieving small goals to get to your end goal, you must visualize those as well.

Below are five steps that you can follow to achieve this visualization:

6. Get yourself to a quiet place and sit down and close your eyes. Start to visualize the final stage of your goals. Imagine that you are experiencing and living the new reality that achieving your goal will bring you, using each of your five senses.
7. Slowly take steps backward from the end goal by visualizing the steps that you would take to achieve your end goal. Imagine the problems you might need to overcome; imagine yourself overcoming them. Picture yourself finding solutions to those problems. Continue visualizing until you reach the moment you are currently living.
8. Next, fast-forward from this moment and imagine which actions helped you overcome your problems.
9. After you finish this visualization, spend a few moments sending your future self some positive vibes and wish them luck on their journey.
10. When you exit the visualization, emotionally detach from the outcome of your goal. One factor that could potentially inhibit you is to having an emotional tie to a particular outcome. Alternatively, try to remain open-

minded, flexible and receptive to whatever is to come on your journey.

You can use visualization using those steps on a daily or weekly basis. Weekly sessions can be as long as 30 minutes, and you can keep your daily sessions shorter, so they are between 5 - 10 minutes. However, be sure that you are using your daily sessions to visualize the next steps on your journey to achieving the goals over the upcoming week. Doing this helps a person to continue making progress towards reaching their goal. After that, you can use your weekly visualizations using the five steps above.

Chapter 10: Motivation

In this chapter, we will look at the all-important and very difficult concept of motivation. First, I will define the term motivation for you, and then we will begin looking at how to find and maintain motivation to keep pursuing your new lifestyle.

What Is Motivation?

Motivation is different for every person. Motivation is different in every area of life, but it is possible to reduce motivation to one single definition.

Motivation is something within a person that drives them towards a wish to change something about their life. These desired changes can be internal (mental, emotional, etc.) or external (in a person's environment). Motivation comes down to wanting to achieve, attain, or accomplish something that you do not have. Motivation combines the desire to change with the desired direction to make a person take action and steps toward the outcomes they want.

Motivation is what helps people accomplish things that they set out to do. For this reason, when trying to accomplish something difficult and challenging, you will search for motivation because it will help you reach your goals.

Now that you understand motivation on a deeper level, we will look at finding and maintaining motivation.

How To Find Motivation

To better understand motivation and how it comes about, we will look at the science behind it.

Some motivation is triggered by needs that you do not even think about, like the need to sustain your life by eating, sleeping, and having connections. Simultaneously, some motivation is triggered by the needs of a psychological nature, such as the need to have a meaningful human connection. To better understand this, we will look at the research of one particular psychologist. Abraham Maslow was a psychologist who specialized in human needs and who came up with a list of human needs that every person seeks to have met. These needs that he researched were broken up into different categories, and within each of these categories are several needs. We will look at these needs below to gain a better understanding of what these categories entail.

Physiological Needs
This category houses the most basic set of needs and includes human needs for survival such as;
- Water
- Air
- Shelter
- Food
- Clothing
- Sleep
- Sex

Safety

This set of needs is the next most basic, but they become a little more abstract in this set than the previous group's physical needs. These needs include;
- Good health
- Employment
- Personal security
- Property
- Resources

Love & Belonging
This set of needs is where it becomes less about what humans need to survive with their basic requirements taken care of and more about those emotional needs. This set of needs includes;
- Family
- Friendship
- Intimacy
- A sense of human connection

Self-Esteem
In this section, this is that set of needs that not everyone can have met in their life, but if you are lucky enough to have these met, you are more privileged than most people on earth. These needs are not extras, as they are still considered human needs, but unfortunately, they are not available to everyone. These needs are;
- Status
- Respect
- Recognition
- Self-esteem
- Freedom
- Strength

Self-Actualization
This section only involves one need, and this single need gives the section its namesake;
- Self-actualization, or the desire to reach one's full potential in every sense of the word.

When it comes to the needs involved in Maslow's findings, you will easily find the motivation to perform tasks that bring you closer to having these needs met. That is because these needs are programmed into every person when they are born, and we spend our lives seeking to fulfill them.

On the other hand, when you are looking to fulfill goals such as; making lots of money, getting a six-pack, or practicing yoga every day for a year, it will be much more difficult to find the motivation to do so. One way around this is to connect your goals to one of the needs in the above lists. For example, say you want to make lots of money. In this case, it may be hard to motivate yourself to pick up an extra job or to stay late at work every night. To combat this, try to connect this want to a human need. In this case, you could say that wanting to make lots of money is connected to a need under the *safety* section, say, property or resources. Alternatively, it could be connected to a need under the *self-esteem* section, say, recognition, or status. It could be connected to any of these needs, or any combination of these needs, depending on the person.

Now, when it comes to the goals that we are discussing in this book, like; losing "x" number of pounds, working out for 30 minutes per day, or cutting out 80% of the sugar from your diet, think about what needs those goals could be connected to. This answer will be personal for you, so take some time to think about this. Doing this on your own will help you find your motivation, as nobody else can find it for you!

How To Maintain Motivation

By examining your motivations, you will be likely to stay on track. By understanding your personal motivating needs for something, you wish to achieve or accomplish, you will likely remember why you began. You will be likely to keep pushing through when things become difficult during the process.

Self-Judgement And How To Overcome It

Self-judgement is something that everybody deals with to some degree. In this section, we will look at how you can take back the reins when it comes to your thoughts and feelings about yourself and how you can begin to re-shift them.

- Be aware

Awareness is the first step that needs to be taken to recognize your inner-critic and reshape it into something less critical and more supportive. Try to pay attention the next time you are feeling distracted, numb, or anxious. Try to identify whose voice is the voice of your inner critic. Try to find the situation where your inner critic awakens. It allows you to dig deep and identify the most vulnerable feelings during situations where your inner critic is awake. These feelings or these situations are likely what your inner critic is trying to protect you from feeling. However, by protecting you, they are holding you back from meeting your full potential. When people have developed unhelpful thinking processes, it is hard to make decisions to benefit their future self because their thoughts create negative emotions that drive away motivation. Some people argue that by simply increasing your willpower, thus overcoming the need for instant gratification, you will fix your situation. This belief, however, is not an effective solution for long-lasting change. In this section, we will look at a variety of ways that you can begin to combat those limiting beliefs and the negative self-talk that goes on in your mind.

- Remind Yourself To Be Positive

As we learned, bad habits are built through many years, and no amount of willpower can handle overcoming that many bad habits in a person's life. Rewiring your brain to minimize the amount of negativity you feel in the first place is a much more efficient method to approach this problem.

- Catch Yourself Thinking According To Your Limiting Beliefs

Often, if the person had just paid attention to their thought process, they would be able to catch themselves before their mind automatically spiraled to a place of complete de-motivation. By catching yourself before you get there, you can prevent yourself from falling into your negative thought patterns, limiting you and holding you back.

- Show Yourself Evidence Against Your Limiting Belief

Showing yourself evidence that supports or doesn't support the thoughts that are on your mind will help you to change your limiting beliefs. Showing yourself evidence can cancel out those negative thinking styles and give yourself the confidence and motivation to overcome any situation.

If a person is stuck in the mindset that they will fail, saying something like, "Oh, I'm going to fail and embarrass myself anyway, so why prepare?" The majority of the time, people of this mindset will choose not to prepare, thus leading to a feeling of failure when they inevitably do not come prepared for success. This mentality further solidifies their limiting belief.

When your inner critic begins to tell you that you can't do a certain thing, or you're not good enough, or you're not worthy enough, simply find evidence within your past life experiences that challenge or discount this belief. Prove your inner critic wrong and show them why holding you back is only going to do more harm than if you failed whatever task you were planning to do. The more you tell your inner critic this, the more they will learn to listen to you and help you in another way that is not just preventing you from doing things.

- Ask For Support From Your Inner Critic

Suppose your inner-critic is telling you that you will embarrass yourself and everyone will laugh at you. In that case, you can first prove it wrong by using evidence-based arguments, negotiate with it to let you try it out, and then ask for its support by saying, "This is a difficult challenge for me, and I want to overcome it. I need you to be by my side, regardless of the outcome." Remember, your inner critic is just another version of yourself. Be kind to it even if it's not kind to you. Showing kindness to yourself is very important in our case.

- Negotiate With Your Limiting Beliefs To Change Them

When you can notice these voices and statements that are going on in your brain according to your limiting beliefs, you can then simply acknowledge them and begin to negotiate with your inner critic. Let them know that you thank them for looking out for you, but you are confident in your ability to make decisions for yourself. You can let them know that even though you may fail and feel embarrassed, it is still better than a lifetime of holding back. Since your inner critic is a part of you, after all, it can listen to reason as long as you allow yourself to be reasoned with.

- Surround Yourself With Positive People

Surrounding yourself with people that can encourage you and foster positivity will also change your inner-critic's opinion. Often, hearing positive compliments from other people hold a heavier weight in the eyes of your inner-critic compared to you telling your inner-critic the same thing. Try spending time with people who support your goals and the changes you are looking to make in your life. It will make your journey a little bit easier.

Limiting beliefs and negative self-talk and negative body-image can lead a person to feel terrible about themselves, often to the point of feeling like they hate themselves. As I mentioned earlier, to make lasting changes, we will work on loving ourselves instead of hating ourselves. By positively seeing your body, because of all of the things it allows you to do, you will begin to make choices with your body's health in mind. Doing this will lead to lasting, positive changes for your physical and mental health.

- Be gentle with yourself.

It is important to be gentle with ourselves because we are usually our own toughest examiner. We look at ourselves very critically, and we often think that nothing we do is good enough. We must be gentle with ourselves to not discourage ourselves, put ourselves down, or make ourselves feel bad about what we are working hard to accomplish. We must remind ourselves that everything in life is a process and does not happen instantly, and we mustn't tell ourselves to "hurry up and succeed," as we often do.

When you fall off track, you must not beat yourself up for this. It is important to be gentle with yourself. Beating yourself up will only cause you to turn into a spiral of negativity and continue to talk down to yourself. Doing this will make you lose motivation and will make you feel like you are a failure. Having this state of mind will make it difficult not to turn to food for comfort. We must avoid this entire process by avoiding beating ourselves up in the first place. If we don't beat ourselves up and instead encourage ourselves, we will not even make ourselves feel the need to find safety. Instead of thinking of how we can't do it, and it is too hard and then needing to turn to food for comfort and a feeling of safety, we will instead talk to ourselves positively and encourage ourselves from within. Instead of making ourselves feel bad, we will instead feel motivated, and we will be even more ready to continue on our journey.

Even if you don't fall off the plan, it is still important to talk to yourself nicely and encourage. We must recognize that changing our behaviors that we have likely been doing for some time is no small feat. We must encourage ourselves just like we would encourage someone else. Think of it like you are talking to a good friend or family member on this journey instead of you. What would you say to them? How would you say it? You would likely be quite gentle and loving in your words. You would likely tell them that they were doing a great job and keeping it up. This example is exactly how you want to speak to yourself from within and the exact types of words and phrases you want to use. If we spoke to our friends the way we speak to ourselves most of the time, they would be quite hurt. Thus, we must remember this when trying to motivate ourselves, and we must be gentle.

Another way to be gentle with yourself is to avoid being too restrictive in the beginning. You must understand that it will be a challenge, and easing into this new lifestyle will be best. Beginning by making small changes and then adding more and more changes as you go will be a good way for your mind and body to get used to the changes. If you dump many changes on yourself too quickly, this will be quite a challenge for your mind and body.

How to Make Your New Lifestyle a Habit

Now that you have learned a wealth of information about intuitive eating, we will look at some strategies that you can use to make these new, healthy choices a habit. Making this a habit will take time, but you will surely find success by employing these strategies.

This section will look at a real-life example of dealing with challenges to demonstrate healthy thinking patterns when it comes to intuitive eating.

Let's say you are trying to focus on healthy eating, and you have had trouble doing so. Maybe you ate a cupcake, or maybe you had a soda at breakfast. From the perspective of the traditional diet mentality, this would become a problem for the diet, which would become a problem in your mind. You would likely be beating yourself up and feeling terrible about the choice you have made.

Let's look at this example in more detail. It is very important to avoid beating yourself up or self-judging for falling off the wagon. Negative self-talk may happen sometimes. What we need to do to combat this is to not focus on the fact that it has happened but on how we are going to deal with and react to it. There are a variety of reactions that a person may have to this type of situation. We will examine the possible reactions and their pros and cons below:

- You may feel as though your progress is ruined and that you might as well begin another time again. This strategy could lead you to go back to your old ways and keep you from trying again for quite some time. This effect could happen many times, over and over again, and each time you slip up, you decide that you might as well give up this time and try again, but each time it ends the same.

- You may fall off your plan and tell yourself that this day is a write-off and that you will begin the next day again. The problem with this method is that continuing the rest of the day as you would have before you decided to make a change will make it so that the next day is like beginning all over again, and it will be very hard to begin again. You may be able to begin the next day again, and it could be fine, but you must be able to motivate yourself if you are going to do this. Knowing that you have fallen off in the past makes it so that you may feel down on yourself and feel as though you can't do it, so beginning again the next day is very important.

- The third option, similar to the previous case, you may fall off, but instead of deciding that the day is a write-off, you tell yourself that the entire week is a write-off, and you then decide that you will pick it up again the next week. This method will be even harder than starting the next day again, as multiple days of eating whatever you like will make it very hard to go back to making the healthy choices again afterward.

- After eating something that you wish you hadn't (and that wasn't a healthy choice), you decide not to eat anything for the rest of the day so that you don't eat too many calories or too much sugar, and decide that the next day you will start over again. Doing this is very difficult on the body as you will be quite hungry by the time the evening rolls around. Instead of forgiving yourself, you are punishing yourself, and it will make it very hard not to reach for chips late at night when you are starving and feeling down.

- The fifth and final option is what you should do in this situation.

This option is the best for success and will make it the most likely to succeed long-term. If you fall off at lunch, let's say, because you are tired and in a rush, and you just grab something from a fast-food restaurant instead of going home for lunch or buying something at the grocery store to eat, this is how we will deal with it. Firstly, you will likely feel like you have failed and may feel quite down about making an unhealthy choice. Now instead of starving for the rest of the day or eating only lettuce for dinner, you will put this slip up at lunch behind you, and you will continue your day as if it never happened. You will eat a healthy dinner as you planned, and you will continue with the plan. You will not wait until tomorrow to begin again; you will continue as you would if you had made that healthy choice at lunch. The key to staying on track can bounce back. The people who can bounce back mentally are the ones who will be most likely to succeed. You will need to maintain a positive mental state and look forward to the rest of the day and the rest of the week in just the same way as you did before you had a slip-up. One bad meal out of the entire week will not ruin all of your progress, and recovering from emotional eating is largely a mental game. It is more mental than anything else, so we must not underestimate our mindset in our success or failure.

Using this type of thinking, you will set yourself up for success and not fall off your plan completely after one slip-up.

Tips For Success

One important way to ensure that these healthy choices stick for good is by changing certain lifestyle aspects. Doing this will reduce the chances of slipping up, which often happens when people eliminate them altogether. For example, you can change the way you approach the grocery store.

When you are entering the grocery store, you must change a few things about how you shop to set yourself up for success. These strategies are especially important when you are just beginning your intuitive eating practice. It will be challenging for you to enter the grocery store and avoid cravings and temptations.

The first thing to keep in mind when grocery shopping for a new diet is to enter with a list. By doing this, you are giving yourself a guide to follow, which will prevent you from picking up things that you are craving or things that you feel like eating at that moment.

One of the biggest things to keep in mind when beginning a new eating practice like intuitive eating is to avoid shopping when you are hungry. Doing this will make you reach for anything and everything that you see. By entering the grocery store when you are satiated or just eaten, you will stick to your list and avoid falling prey to temptations.

If you treat your grocery shopping experience like a treasure hunt, you will be able to cross things off of the list one at a time without venturing to the parts of the grocery store that will prove to be a challenge for you to resist. If you are making healthy eating choices, you will likely be spending most of your time at the perimeter of the grocery store. This location is where the whole, plant-based foods are located. By doing this and entering with a list, you will avoid the middle aisles where the processed, high-sugar temptation foods are all kept.

Having a plan is key when it comes to learning new habits and employing a new lifestyle. This plan can be as detailed as you wish, or it can simply come in the form of a general overview. I recommend you start with a more detailed plan in the beginning as you ease into things.

As everyone is different, you may be the type of person who likes lots of lists and plans, or you may be the type of person who doesn't, but for everyone, beginning with a plan and following it closely for the first little while is best. For example, this plan can include; what you will focus on each week, what you will reduce your intake of, and what you will try to achieve in terms of the mental work involved.

Once you have come up with a general plan for your new lifestyle and how you want it to look, you can begin laying out more specific plans.

Planning your meals will make it much easier for you when you get home from work or when you wake up tired in the morning and need to pack something for your lunch.

You can plan your meals out a week in advance, two weeks, or even a month if you wish. You can post this up on your fridge, and each day you will know exactly what you are eating, with no thinking required. This way, there won't be a chance for you to consider ordering a pizza or heating up some chicken fingers because you will already know exactly what you will make. By approaching your new style of eating in this way, you can make this transition easier on yourself and ensure success every step of the way.

Conclusion

Weight loss is much more than simply eating vegetables and going to the gym. This book taught you that weight loss involves much deeper concepts and much harder work than just this.

This book took a deep dive into various topics surrounding the psychology of body image, weight loss, and motivation. We looked at how you can control your internal self to accomplish anything and achieve your goals. This book aimed to equip you with the tools you need to control your life and change your body for the better. Through reading this book, I hope that you found some peace and a sense of compassion for yourself, as bringing about change is not an easy task.

We began by learning about some of the situations and causes that most often lead people to become overweight by looking at the connection between your mind and your physical body. We looked at some strategies for getting in touch with your emotions and feelings to determine what led you to where you currently are. We then learned about hypnosis and how it can help you make changes in your life. Now that you are equipped with various hypnosis techniques, you can begin practicing them in your daily life. Hypnosis is an invaluable tool for weight loss, and now that you have reached the end of this book, you are ready to take it into your own hands.

After addressing the psychological side of weight loss and body image, we learned about the science of weight loss, weight loss techniques, diets, and exercise. We looked at how you can plan around your lifestyle to ensure success. Finally, we looked at how to put everything we learned together in the form of a plan and how to deal with inevitable challenges or setbacks that you may face along the way.

It is important to remember that weight loss, a change of mind, or a change in rooted behaviors do not happen in one day or even in one week. The key to making any sort of change that will last in your life is consistency. You must be consistent in your hypnosis practice, diet, change of behaviors, and every component of your new lifestyle to see changes. If, for some reason, you slip up, remind yourself that you are not a failure and continue where you left off. This reminder will be the key to maintaining consistency and make changes in your life.

I hope that through reading this book, you have developed a deeper knowledge of how you can begin to change your life in much deeper ways than losing weight, but by also acknowledging and tackling the underlying causes of your unhappiness. By doing the hard work that this book helps you to realize, you can find lasting weight loss instead of a fluctuating number on the scale.

If you take one thing from this book, let it be the idea that you and your body must work as one. Do not fight with your mind or body, but instead work with it, and you will find harmony.

I wish you luck in your journey, and I hope that you continue to pursue lasting change.

Printed in Great Britain
by Amazon